Out of Your Comfort Zone

"I seriously pushed my boundaries and found great inspiration from reading *Mind Body Diabetes* and then reading Emma's second book *Out of Your Comfort Zone*. I found it a powerful and enlightening read in so many ways, the perfect resource taking me to new and exciting heights with my life in general. A truly excellent book for whatever stage of life you're at, with whatever fears or holdbacks you may have."

—JO BERRY, peace activist, public speaker,
and conflict resolution consultant

"Seeing Dr Em and applying everything in this book, I've learned how to step out of my comfort zone and seriously break boundaries to experience an amazing life that was once unimaginable, given my severe traumatic anxiety. From being told I'd always be on antidepressants to now being medication-free, I'm a happy, healthy, and successful 23-year-old. Thank you so much. A brilliant read encapsulating everything!"

—JASMINE DOUGHTY, civil servant and
positive change advocate

"Having experienced life at my lowest ebb, to the extent I was ready to end it all, I can say 100 per cent that Em made an enormous difference in the way I saw life. Without all her help—basically everything she's put in this book—and her natural manner to add a certain sense of humour and solution in even the darkest times, I would have been pushed over the edge. Thanks to all our work I'm a totally different person from that time and for sure out of my comfort zone, pushing new boundaries like you wouldn't believe! Thank you so much."

—VINCENT SHAY, ex-military personnel,
outdoor pursuits trainer, and youth leader

D0992715

OUT
OF **YOUR COMFORT ZONE**

BREAKING BOUNDARIES FOR
A LIFE BEYOND LIMITS

EMMA MARDLIN, Ph.D.

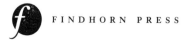

FINDHORN PRESS

Findhorn Press
One Park Street
Rochester, Vermont 05767
www.findhornpress.com

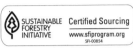

Text stock is SFI certified

Findhorn Press is a division of Inner Traditions International

Disclaimer
The information in this book is given in good faith and is neither intended to diagnose any physical or mental condition nor to serve as a substitute for informed medical advice or care. Please contact your health professional for medical advice and treatment. Neither author nor publisher can be held liable by any person for any loss or damage whatsoever which may arise from the use of this book or any of the information therein.

Cataloging-in-Publication Data for this title is available from the Library of Congress

ISBN 978-1-62055-824-9 (print)
ISBN 978-1-62055-825-6 (ebook)

Printed and bound in the United States by Lake Book Manufacturing, Inc. The text stock is SFI certified. The Sustainable Forestry Initiative® program promotes sustainable forest management.

10 9 8 7 6 5 4 3 2 1

Edited by Jacqui Lewis
Text design and layout by Geoff Green Book Design
This book was typeset in Utopia
Illustrations by Emma Mardlin, except for p. 27: Bing Images/Artist Istvan Orosz

To send correspondence to the author of this book, mail a first-class letter to the author c/o Inner Traditions • Bear & Company, One Park Street, Rochester, VT 05767, USA and we will forward the communication, or contact the author directly at www.dr-em.co.uk

To my mum, Clare,
who has always pushed her own boundaries in amazing ways, and is
continually encouraging my sister and me to do the same.

To my sister, Francesca, incredibly pushing a very personal comfort
zone in having her first baby this year –
a massive congratulations to
Chess, Andy and Maddison Alexandra Dutton,
Born 5 October 2018!

Enormous thanks to

My partner, and close family and friends, who continue to inspire and encourage me in various ways, particularly those named throughout this book.

Valuentis Limited for their support in getting my questionnaires online to share with the rest of the world. All my clients, delegates, students and readers, who continue to push their own boundaries in amazing ways, achieving phenomenal results.

My personal healthcare team, who allow me the space and discretion to continually push my own medical boundaries and research.

CONTENTS

PUSHING PERSONAL BOUNDARIES

"It's the best way to test yourself. Have fun and push boundaries."

Richard Branson

Happily using the past tense, and without trying to sound too dramatic, I've quite literally stared death in the face a good few times, and had to confront issues I was petrified of when facing some things I'd never even contemplated.

Being told I was going blind, for one. Or finding myself in a critical medical situation mid-flight at high altitude over a war zone, with essential work commitments to deliver the next morning in a foreign country. Not to mention the many business bombshells and life curveballs along the way that have pushed me well outside my personal comfort zone.

From as young an age as I can remember my mum has encouraged my sister and me to do the things we were most scared to do. Essentially, she was encouraging us to push out of our comfort zones, despite us usually making a fuss and wanting to run a mile! Although to be fair to my sister and me, this did include removing spiders from the bath, riding the biggest roller coasters, stroking every creepy-looking animal in the zoo and confronting bullies, as well as speaking to people we'd usually hide from, ordering from the menu for ourselves and – wait for it – even meeting the sullen bank manager by ourselves to start our kids' saver accounts . . . you name it, we had to do it!

My mum is in no way a horrible mum (although we did try threatening her with Childline a few times for making us do all the things we feared). She is in fact a brilliant mum and incredibly smart too. By actively encouraging us from the off to smash right through any comfort zones, break our boundaries and develop new resources, she raised two very resilient girls.

And now I know all too well that one of the core principles of successfully pushing through your comfort zone is to do the very things that scare you by putting yourself in a space where you have little other choice. In the words of Richard Branson, "Screw it, just do it"!

However, I also know it's not always that simple as we develop and go through life to remain unaffected by the various traumas and curveballs that can come hurtling our way. They can leave a nasty dent to the head that seems to imprint on the mind, often leaving a lasting impression.

Although I'm a resilient character, I'm definitely not infallible when it comes to fear. Professionally in all I do, coupled with, in my personal life, managing two chronic conditions as well as life and business in general, I deal with fear in one way or another pretty much daily . . . so one might say I've gone the extra mile, having tried and tested everything I write about, develop and do. I'm also no stranger to having to step out of my comfort zone and push my own boundaries to the extreme, as my work and research involves the full reversal of Type 1 diabetes, which has never before been done in this way and is often misunderstood. So, as I'm the primary lab rat most days, and seriously having to practise what I preach, it puts me to the test!

When it comes to personal experience of facing fear, I've certainly been around the block a few times, which has enabled me to develop experientially most of the resources you'll find in this book.

Although, thanks to my mum, my natural instinct is to just get on with things whether I feel the fear or not, I've equally been confronted with outright fears where such an approach hasn't been possible. And we're all different in the fears we experience and the ways in which we can deal with them. Hence the book takes a multi-pronged approach to stepping outside comfort zones.

Here, from my personal experience, are two examples of different kinds of fears, the different kinds of situations from which they arose and the different kinds of resilience and resources needed to tackle them.

Since I was very small I've never liked heights, and over time this only ever got worse by developing into a full-blown, irrational fear (acrophobia). This got so out of hand that:

I missed out on going up the Eiffel Tower with friends.

I missed seminars at university because they had been moved to the top floor of a tower building and despite my best attempts I just froze on the stairs. I had a lot of notes to catch up on!

I completely ruined my birthday surprise, a concert, by sitting petrified throughout in the gods – I literally didn't move from beginning to end and spent the whole time planning how I was going to get down from what seemed like the ceiling without a fuss – thank goodness for the very tall man in front of me shielding me from the view!

On one holiday I held everyone up at the end of a jungle assault course because I hadn't realized that in order to complete it you had to walk across a stupidly high rope bridge. Despite an irate German kid pushing me from behind and shouting obscenities at me to get on with it, I had to run the whole course backwards, as my only other option to escape.

Although I knew all too well I needed to do something about this (aside from ensuring no one booked me concert tickets ever again!) for a while I got by just planning things accordingly– basically I used an avoidance strategy. That worked well . . .

Up to a point, of course! One day I suddenly found myself in a tricky situation, and it was only then that something changed inside me.

As part of my work, I lecture and train abroad in hotel conference rooms and colleges which are usually on the first floor. However, on one occasion I hadn't been told where exactly the training session was going to be and only found out when I arrived that everyone was already there waiting in the training room which was on the top floor of (you've guessed it) a lovely great big high-rise hotel. I was contracted to do this work, so I couldn't even enlist my partner to do it on my behalf, and there would be serious repercussions if I suddenly cancelled the course. So, with my adrenaline pumping, I literally had no choice in the matter but to confront my fear this time. Even the elevator only went so far, so I had to negotiate some horrible stairs too.

I did make it to the top (albeit very breathlessly and feeling dreadful) and straight into the training room. By the end of the day I had become accustomed to being so high up, to the point where I dared myself to go onto the balcony to look outside. I saw the beautiful views I had been missing out on, as well as realizing that I was actually OK, just like everyone else.

So, through having an overriding intention for doing something that was greater than the very thing I was petrified of, as well as being forced to face my once-crippling fear, I had overcome it.

My younger sister, Francesca, had an intense (and I don't mean that lightly) fear of hospitals, ambulances and anything clinical or medical in nature. She wouldn't even drive past a hospital or behind an ambulance. Its formal name is nosocomephobia and it is actually quite a common phobia – U.S President Richard Nixon was a sufferer and his famous remark "If I go to a hospital, I'm fairly sure I won't come out of it alive" probably resonates with quite a few people.

However, in approximately 2008 this fear was majorly put to the test. I was in a serious coma in hospital and my family had been told that I might not wake up, or that I could have brain damage. It took some time for my sister to manage to come to the hospital, and then it was only for a flying visit only when I was recovering in a private room. This major event made her realize that she needed – and wanted – to do something about her phobia.

So we had to look at the root cause, pertaining to her significant memory of a hospital. This related to a family trauma that she witnessed when she was only four years old, in her "imprint" period of development, when memories imprint on our minds and shape our deep beliefs, core values and personality (this is discussed in more detail later).

It was a deep and intense experience and required her to work with some equally intense but incredibly powerful techniques. Resilient as ever, my sister battled on until she had totally overcome her phobia. Then ten years later in March 2018 she announced that she was expecting her first baby, something that because of the impending medical involvement, her phobia had once meant was unthinkable for her.

So by now you'll have gathered that there are many powerful ways to deal with and release all kinds of fear and countless types of phobias. And it's important too to recognize that, no matter how big or small or how crazy you may think these fears, phobias and life limitations are, if they matter to you, they matter – because ultimately they are the fears that are holding you back from stepping outside your comfort zone and breaking your personal boundaries to live a life beyond limits and be all that you can be.

The great news is that, as you have heard from me and my sister's stories, there's so much you can do to work on all kinds of fears, phobias or limitations.

The aim of *Out of Your Comfort Zone* is to show you how you can break your own boundaries, discover new boundaries that you didn't even know you had and successfully confront fear, as well as release anxiety and build indestructible resilience to realize a new, exciting life beyond limits. It is enriched by many of the neat tricks, psychological techniques and exciting unorthodox approaches that I regularly use in my practice to help people overcome anything – from phobias to outright traumas and intense anxiety – that stops them achieving everything they otherwise could. A complete resource guide to refer to at will, whenever needed.

On that note, enjoy your personal journey, have fun – and go for it, in every way you can!

CHAPTER ONE

THE ZONE TEST: DETERMINING YOUR COMFORT ZONE LEVEL RIGHT NOW

D espite all of us having different comfort zones for different reasons, one thing's for sure: we all have them, whether pertaining to the most intense of fears and anxieties, deeply buried limitations or just downright quirky phobias. This book is all about assisting you with breaking your personal comfort zone, losing those associated fears, anxieties and limitations. Really pushing boundaries and going beyond to master a different level of thinking that can give you the life you really want!

So, before we seriously get started, it will be useful to take the Zone Test to establish your current comfort zone and highlight what aspects of life might be holding you back; right from the obvious things to the things you may not be consciously aware of. This will provide you with a personal platform to work from, and a greater sense of self-awareness to evolve.

The Zone Test appears at the end of the book too, so that you can retake it, compare your scores from now and then, and also see the results of your progress. It will also highlight any areas you feel you'd like or you need to strengthen.

> *"I learned that courage was not the absence of fear but the triumph over it."*
>
> Nelson Mandela

Using this introspective quiz, you will be able to see which zone you fall into and look at the areas in your life you can positively think differently about and change in order to push yourself forward to reach zone zero. This is the point at which you no longer have boundaries or irrational fears – just challenges that you know you'll quite easily smash through as and when you need to, leaving you to enjoy a fulfilled and exhilarating life.

It's important to note that in answering the following questions, there are no right or wrong answers, just your individual preferences; these indicate to what extent you display the common psychological attributes associated with pushing personal boundaries and stepping outside common comfort zones to live your life to the full and achieve everything you desire.

You can also read more in depth about what each question and answer represent. Do this after completing the test so that it does not influence your answers. It will help you to further understand your answers, providing you with greater insight about your current inner self so that you can get the maximum value out of this book.

As this test is a measurement tool for you and your own personal development, you'll get the most out of it if you answer the questions as honestly and quickly as possible.

Remember these questions are generic and based on self-analysis; therefore the results are not to be read as any kind of formal psychological measure, but rather as an indication of your current comfort zone and zone description where you are at in your life.

You can take The Zone Test™ online and receive your score and zone instantly: go to https://zonetest.questionpro.com

Otherwise, read on and take the test below.

> *"The fears we don't face become our limits."*
>
> Robin Sharma

The Zone Test

Choose the option most applicable to you.

Q1. The last time I did something that scared me, or I made a bold decision, for personal growth, was:

    a. Can't really remember
    b. Within the last month
    c. Within the last year
    d. Within the last six months

Q2. If I am faced with a situation that involves being presented with the opportunity to do something that really makes me feel uncomfortable, I will:

    a. Avoid the situation entirely
    b. Purposely put myself forward
    c. Find an excuse to just avoid doing the thing I don't like
    d. Decide I'll do it if I absolutely have to

Q3. I implicitly trust my intuition:

    a. Rarely
    b. Always
    c. Occasionally
    d. Usually

Q4. Others think of me as different or unconventional:

    a. Never
    b. Always
    c. Perhaps
    d. Usually

Q5. I find making changes challenging to do:

    a. Always
    b. Never
    c. Usually
    d. Occasionally

Q6. Scenario: I am the CEO of a business and have to make the difficult decision about which one of two employees to let go. One is my sibling, good at their job albeit not one of the best, but I know that their personal situation leaves them critically reliant on this job. The other employee is very good at their job with an impeccable employment record.
    I would favour the family member:

    a. Always
    b. Occasionally
    c. Usually
    d. Never

Q7. When there's a problem I am calm and easily see many solutions:

   a. Never
   b. Always
   c. Occasionally
   d. Usually

Q8. On a given project someone has to be in control, so the person with the most knowledge should lead, even if that person is not me:

   a. Never
   b. Usually
   c. Occasionally
   d. Always

Q9. In my life, I know I have everything I need to fully take care of myself; I believe I am always responsible for everything that happens in my life, even if something isn't my fault:

   a. Never
   b. Always
   c. Occasionally
   d. Usually

Q10. I change my profile picture on social media accounts such as Whats-App, Facebook, Twitter and Instagram:

   a. Very often
   b. Occasionally
   c. Quite often
   d. Never

Q11. I am currently doing everything I can do, irrespective of obstacles or challenges, to lead the life I want:

   a. Never
   b. Always
   c. Occasionally
   d. Usually

Q12. I have no problem with open-ended (non-specific) plans that fit within a general framework:

    a. Never
    b. Always
    c. Occasionally
    d. Usually

Q13. I do what I do because I have to and I see little alternative:

    a. Always
    b. Never
    c. Occasionally
    d. Usually

Q14. I have taken part in some of the following sports/activities before – skydiving, bungee jumping, scuba/shark diving, paragliding, flying/piloting yourself, climbing a mountain or volcano, paintballing, motor racing, speedboating, skiing, big theme-park rides/roller coasters or similar:

    a. Never
    b. Absolutely and I do whenever I can
    c. Just not interested
    d. Tried but never again

Q15. If there's something I really want in life, I always find a way to do it or get it. I have my goals and I know I will achieve them:

    a. Never
    b. Always
    c. Occasionally
    d. Usually

Q16. I can't start new projects that I feel I have little experience in, qualifications or funds for:

    a. Always
    b. Never
    c. Usually
    d. Occasionally

Q17. I have a profound anxiety, fear or phobia that prevents me from enjoying the things I would like to do or could be doing:

    a. True

    b. In the past and overcome

    c. Sometimes

    d. Never

Q18. I don't like to be around indecisive people:

    a. Very true

    b. Occasionally true

    c. Usually true

    d. False

Q19. I like to visit places I've never been before:

    a. Never

    b. Always

    c. Occasionally

    d. Usually

Q20. I feel uncomfortable with lack of routine, unfamiliar situations and doing things I don't usually do:

    a. Always

    b. Never

    c. Occasionally

    d. Usually

Q21. I play games and sports for fun and fitness, not just for the sake of winning (excluding playing professionally):

    a. Never

    b. Always

    c. Occasionally

    d. Usually

Q22. I won't try or say things that others haven't before me:

    a. Always

    b. Never

    c. Usually

    d. Occasionally

Q23. If I have an issue about something that needs dealing with, I directly confront it as soon as possible:

    a. Never
    b. Always
    c. Occasionally
    d. Usually

Q24. If I don't always know the answer for sure it won't stop me answering; I say what I think is best and move on:

    a. Never
    b. Always
    c. Occasionally
    d. Usually

Q25. I won't do certain things if I potentially make a fool of myself:

    a. Always
    b. Never
    c. Usually
    d. Occasionally

For the following statements, choose true or false.

Q26. If my doctor strongly recommends something to me or simply assumes I will follow their advice over a serious matter, but I disagree, I am adamant in going with my own decision:

    a. True
    b. False

Q27. I never usually worry about my mistakes:

    a. True
    b. False

Q28. If there's something I really want/need, such as starting a business or charity, having children, a personal mission, moving abroad, changing or starting a new job or career, further education/qualifications, writing a book, surgery, treatment, therapy or anything else relevant to me, I never find reasons to put it off:

    a. True
    b. False

Q29. I have successfully completed a profound, life-changing, personal mission of mine:

    a. True

    c. False

Q30. If something has to be completed under time pressure I don't usually find it a problem and in fact tend to thrive under the pressure:

    a. True

    b. False

Q31. I know I am good at what I do, and I love who I am. I don't need to justify it regardless of what people think of me:

    a. True

    b. False

The Answers and Zones

Points for your answers to questions 1 to 25:

    a = 1 point

    b = 4 points

    c = 2 points

    d = 3 points

Points for your answers to questions 26 to 31:

    a. True = 1 point

    b. False = 0 points

Below see a brief explanation of what each question is about:

Q1. General personality/life direction and personal boundaries

Q2. Self-motivation to push oneself/putting yourself in the space

Q3. Self-awareness, self-consciousness, confidence and self-reliance

Q4. Self-assurance/-awareness/thinking style

Q5. Flexibility and resistance to change

Q6. Emotional reasoning and the need to be liked

Q7. Flexible/creative thinking, confidence, problem-solving, pressure

Q8. Pragmatism, control, pride and results-orientation

Q9. Self-responsibility, self-reliance, resourcefulness, confidence, independence; need for certainty

Q10. Seeking social approval – need for recognition, to be liked, fit in with popular culture, personal insecurities, comparing/competing with others to appear "good enough"/the need to assert.

Q11. Ambition and seeing solutions, not problems

Q12. Flexibility, believing in oneself and trusting the process of life

Q13. Seizing opportunity, acting out of possibility or necessity, determination and subjugation

Q14. Liking the feeling of adrenaline and thrill-seeking

Q15. Determination, knowing outcome and strength of positive belief system

Q16. Fear of failure or making mistakes

Q17. Existing fear measurement

Q18. Control and taking charge

Q19. Adventure and dealing with uncertainty

Q20. Fear of the unknown, need for safety and security

Q21. Fear of failure and humiliation – ability to see the bigger picture

Q22. Experimentation and control

Q23. Assertiveness and courage

Q24. Independent thought and fear of mistakes

Q25. Inhibitions

Q26. Authority, independent thought, self-belief and confidence

Q27. Self-confidence, anxiety levels and decision-making

Q28. Subconscious fears

Q29. Current position and expectations

Q30. Putting pressure on oneself and thinking style

Q31. Judgement

Zone Test Scores

The Comfy Zone (<50)

You like your comfort zone: you are more likely to be averse to risk, more fearful of making mistakes and taking chances, and resistant to change. You tend to be a more cautious, anxious person when it comes to pushing boundaries and would rather play safe and content than risk anything greater; therefore you settle more easily for things. Perhaps you have been awaiting the right opportunity to change how you feel and are ready to take this opportunity to unleash a transformed, forward-focused you who feels they now deserve to have everything they have only ever previously dreamed about. If one person can do it, so can you and this book will provide you with the right support, mindset and practical resources to do just that. Now you can turn those dreams into a realistic plan.

The Exploring Zone (51–74)

You are likely warming up for action, looking to increase confidence and let go of anxieties, judgement and emotional reasoning; possibly with a person in mind who you'd like to be, or the life you'd like to have. You seem to have an average level of fears and anxieties but are mostly aware of them and want to get rid. You mainly need to let go of inhibitions and the need for control. You do like to gently stretch yourself and try new experiences, but in a safe space to minimize risk and the chances of mistakes or failure. You will find the resilience-builders a great help and positive step forward to successfully transition through zones to reach where you want to be.

The Break-Out Zone (75–100)

You are already breaking out. Displaying or feeling ready for new levels of thinking and that final push to take you to zone zero. You exhibit all the traits of a zone-zero personality but need to be more congruent and wholly consistent in them with full conviction and an unshakable self-belief.

You are certainly a risk-taker who enjoys a good challenge. You are generally pretty fearless about failure or making mistakes; however, slight trepidation over this and a little self-doubt can sometimes hold you back from really going for it and taking advantage of more opportunities with likely success. You'd greatly benefit from learning to trust more in the process of life as well as yourself. Enhancing your intuition even further will help with this too. You are not too concerned about the judgement of others, but are more than aware of it, which may occasionally contribute to delaying your personal progress.

Generally, you are a bold, thrill-seeking person who dares to be different. You are generally very comfortable in taking risks and do like to challenge your own comfort zone. The later chapters of this book in particular will be a great tool in providing you with that final push.

Zone Zero (101 +)

Congratulations; you're already there! Perhaps you're looking for a few reminders of who you really are if you're feeling a little off form for whatever reason? Otherwise you're unlikely to have taken this test or found it in the first place (be this consciously or subconsciously and via whatever unlikely channel – you'll know there's a reason!).

This happens to us all and you'll find all you need in this book, whether a positive support to reignite your fuse or that prompt to take you to another level. Chapter Eight will be of particular interest and all you need just now.

The Zone Chart

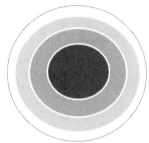

Dark Grey – The Comfy Zone
Grey – The Exploring Zone
Light Grey – Break-Out Zone
White – The Uncomfortable and Boundary
        Pushing Stages
No Boundaries – Zone Zero

Whatever stage you may be at in terms of your current comfort zone level, when transitioning between any level, there's always an uncomfortable and boundary pushing stage that we must all push through and overcome – this is depicted as the white rings on the chart above. This stage is where the real positive change happens, allowing us to evolve and transition to new heights. As the zone colours become lighter, although present in any level, this transitioning becomes far less challenging as we become more accustomed to the elements required to push our boundaries.

This journey of progression forms our personal evolution and is the point at which we really learn and transition into who and what we ultimately want to be, to reach total fulfilment. It can also be useful to further ask yourself:

- Why you gave the answers you did and what specifically you were referring to – noting these points down now can also make for an even more interesting comparison when you check your progress at the end of the book.
- Finally, did you discover anything new about yourself from thinking through the questions?
- Are you ready to expand your comfort zone to where you want to go, learn more about yourself or simply reignite a new fresh purpose to keep things exciting and see just how far you can go with limitless boundaries and thinking?

"Who would you be and what would you have,
if you had no comfort zone?"

CHAPTER TWO

WHAT'S THE BIG IDEA?

When was the last time you did something that scared you; the last time you really put yourself to the test, took a risk and pushed your boundaries such that you bulldozed right through them? Essentially, when was the last time you stepped outside of your comfort zone and used it to make positive change to hurtle yourself forward in life?

Conversely, have you ever asked yourself "What didn't I do because I decided to stay within the confines of my comfort zone? If I had decided otherwise, what could I have achieved?"

Whenever and whatever your answer may be, if you've ever successfully confronted and overcome a particular fear of doing something, it's a fair bet that you felt an overwhelming sense of freedom, total liberation, self-worth and fulfilling satisfaction. A pretty awesome feeling, I'm sure you'll agree!

Well, just for a few moments, imagine feeling like this all the time. That amazing feeling when you've overcome something, smashed right through your boundaries and consequently feel unstoppable; as if there's now nothing in the world to prevent you from doing and getting everything you want. A new way of thinking that provides you with a true sense of liberation; a breath of freedom allowing you to fully take in life. Now imagine being able to feel this way permanently – and know that if you really want to, you're now going to powerfully learn how.

There are of course many reasons that have prevented us and will continue to regularly try to prevent us from even getting so far as stepping outside our comfort zone to experience those exhilarating feelings. However, that's one of the main aims of this book: to provide the resources to rip them out of the way and remove them for good, leaving absolutely nothing in your way.

The main idea behind this book is "Daring to be Different": thinking and approaching things differently for very different results; backed up practically by the approach of "Doing something daily that challenges you" to build up a tenacious resilience. The latter being a brilliant approach that is specifically promoted by a business associate and good friend of mine, Anthony Hall, as "Do Something Every Day That Scares You". The idea is to challenge yourself, and positively embrace fear in order to ultimately confront and conquer the biggest demons that are currently holding you back or that life may one day randomly surprise you with.

Although the things potentially holding you back will vary enormously from seemingly minor to major, one thing that's for sure is that, whatever your preventing factor may be, whatever is really holding you back from everything you want will pertain to a fear (or other derived negative emotion) in one form or another.

In which case, we all have essentially two choices:

1. Bottle it and stay comfortable in the "sameness" for a lifetime.
2. Dare to be different, think differently, create change, step outside your zone and break some boundaries.

With three main ways to implement the second option:

1. Screw it, just do it.
2. Build up resilience, utilize specific resources and put yourself in the space.
3. Extract the core root, change your mindset and determine an amazing life.

This book shares with you everything necessary to successfully implement all three options, equipping you with all that's needed to conquer your fears and limitations, big or small and from the physically tangible to the purely psychological. Everything you need is integrated to allow you to go forth and achieve everything you can, in every context you wish.

There are plenty of behavioural psychologists and other healthcare professionals who will gladly tell you that there are no magic words that can be said to change the way we feel about being anxious and feeling uneasy or scared. They believe instead that these feelings can only be overcome by changing the way we behave – hence they are advocates of the "Screw it, just do it" or "Do Something Every Day That Scares You" philosophy. In a nutshell, they're saying that, in order to get over an anxious feeling or profound fear, we must simply confront it – which naturally means learning to deal with what makes us feel uncomfortable, inevitably pushing us outside of our comfort zone.

Certainly, this is all true, BUT only to a degree, because if it was that easy, wouldn't we all just confront our fears and be done with it?

We first have to change how we think in order to change how we feel because it's the thinking part that comprises all the specific neurochemicals and pathways that initially create the irrational fear; it is the subsequent feeling or emotion generated that ultimately changes how we behave and therefore the results we get.

So actually, there are some very powerful words and techniques that can allow you to release unnecessary pre-anxiety; and you may need to address this first, prior to confronting your primary fear and major positive change.

After all, we mustn't overlook change itself, because everything that comes with stepping outside your comfort zone and breaking boundaries inevitably involves creating an exciting new reality, a new you who attracts completely different results; and for some people, such change can be just as scary as confronting the initial fear itself.

So, the approach of applying resilience-builders and addressing the root cause techniques first will subsequently enable you to recognize and take action to confront your fears, remove limitations and break your comfort zone in the first place. This will establish your ability to confront your fear by looking back on having successfully conquered it rather than applying these techniques in order to conquer your fear in a more reactive sense.

And when you are ready to test it, that which was once a problem and an overwhelming fear will no longer be a problem at all. I refer to this as a "real" problem blowout.

Love him or loathe him, there's no greater current example of this than Donald Trump himself being inaugurated as the U.S. President. Quite simply, he believed he would be President, he said he would be, and he is! There are so many ways to release and conquer those irrational fears that impede your life journey and insist on holding you back from reaching your full potential; after all, they're seldom a real or even tangible threat.

> *"We do not fear the unknown. We fear what we think we know about the unknown."*
>
> Teal Swan

For example, when it comes to some universal fears, did you know that:

- Fear of flying, aerophobia – You're more likely to become a professional athlete or be in a car accident than be involved in a plane crash.
- Fear of thunder and lightning, astraphobia – Thunder is not regarded as particularly dangerous and it's very rare to be struck by lightning since up to 90 per cent of the lightning travels from cloud to cloud rather than reaching the ground.
- Fear of spiders, arachnophobia – Only 12 out of 40,000 species of spiders can cause serious harm to adult humans.
- Fear of the dentist, dentophobia – Modern dental techniques such as air abrasion have replaced many traumatic dental treatments of the past.
- Not to mention, regarding any fear of particular things harming you, you'll discover new scientific quantum ways of thinking later in the book to ensure you can avoid this.
- There are only two "real" fears that we are actually born with: fear of falling (often confused with fear of heights) and fear of loud noises. Meaning everything else we fear is a story that we have somehow created and that we hold on to in our minds.

Fears are therefore simply stories that we tell ourselves, and can be conveniently referred to as False Evidence Appearing Real.

That's why one of the key principles here is to help you to build up resilience and deal with anything that scares you – big or small; whatever holds you back in life. It will help you to recognize the root and extract the fear for good.

In making you step out of your comfort zone, it will make you think deeply about your life and push your personal boundaries.

How easy is it to go on in life just being content with staying all cosy in a nice safe comfort zone?

Well, I'm sure you'll agree it's far too easy! However, comfort zones can equally prove pretty "hamster wheelish", creating a boring monotony that ultimately prevents us from growing and developing personally, socially and professionally; we could be fulfilling goals we may have once deemed possible, but instead if we stay too cosy we come to accept them dwindling away or – even worse – we just give up on them.

Following the process of incrementally breaking out of your comfort zone will help you to start seeing life differently; as more of an adventure.

So much so that when you change how you see your life, you will find your-self experiencing a whole new world.

Essentially, you'll be choosing to take control of your mind and therefore your life. In doing so you'll begin to determine your own internal reality, which will then change your external reality – how you experience the world and how life treats you in response; basically, the results you get, as opposed to letting the outside world determine how you feel on the inside, which all too often becomes a self-defeating vicious circle. The point when we all decide to take full responsibility for ourselves and become aware and accepting of the fact that we are the ones who can influence where we want to go in life, is the moment when we create the biggest change possible! And thus the aim of this book is to share with you how to positively do that, such that the concept of a comfort zone will soon become a thing of the past.

Working through this process will therefore help you build up a certain resilience whereby you won't fear exploring new frontiers, or the things that you were once scared to confront, like fear of the unknown, fear of failure or fear of change.

So, this book is also about encouraging a mindset that knows no bounds, seeks excitement in the unknown and in change and sees failure as merely a positive lesson to push forward or do it better next time round.

All too often it can take something exceptionally drastic in life for people to realize they need, or indeed want, to change. However, by applying all the concepts in this book, you won't have to wait for this to happen. You can start by taking small steps today to make big strides and major positive changes thereafter, achieving everything you want and desire.

You can make one change instantly by thinking about thinking. If you start to see things differently, things will begin to look different and you'll soon feel like a whole new you.

Now notice, what's the first thing you "feel", when looking at each image:

 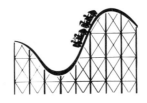 

Dread? Fear? Nerves? Excitement? Fun? Challenge?

What's interesting with this question is that, even though everyone is looking at and talking about exactly the same image or idea, people will always give different answers for different reasons.

Pretty much as you could have two people riding a roller coaster, essentially doing exactly the same thing, yet one person may be shaking with fear and the other laughing with excitement and anticipation.

Similarly, with two people talking to a roomful of 200 people, one of them could be enjoying and embracing it while the other is feeling sick with nerves and stuttering their way through it.

So clearly no two experiences are ever the same, which tells us one thing: Everything is in the mind!

The exciting part of this revelation is that fear is most often an intangible creation of our own thoughts! We can take this even further and surmise that fear is never really the problem – fear is just the reaction. A manifestation of our thoughts connected to the trigger, which is the only real problem.

So, if one person can be fearless about the very same thing that scares you witless . . . you can lose any fear when applying the right mindset!

The Staple Seven to Successful Results

These seven primciples keep you focused on achieving successful results.

1. **Awareness that our internal reality is what creates our external results**
   - If we have a negative, fearful or constantly cynical mindset that forms our individual, internal reality in our head, we'll externally experience results in line with this thinking. For example, if we're fearful, we won't do certain things and therefore won't move forward. Similarly, if you're deep-down negative about something, you're unlikely to experience positive results regarding it.
   - Choose to create a positive internal reality instead (that is, the stories you tell yourself and how things play out in your own head – how you perceive and see things, therefore how you think and feel about life). This then causes your external reality (the outside world) to change accordingly. There is more specific detail about this in Chapter Eight.
   - In a nutshell, this is about knowing you can take control rather than merely responding and reacting to your external world and letting that determine your internal state and entire life.

- This is exciting stuff, and the more you can appreciate and apply it, the better results you'll always get; you will experience positive change in your life, as fully explained in Chapters Six and Eight.

2. A positive focus and limited "refractory period"

There are always curveballs in life and naturally plenty of obstacles to challenge us, but there's a lot of truth in the cliché "What doesn't kill you makes you stronger" – or at least there can be if you have the right mindset and learn to automatically look at things differently. Quite simply, although we all need to express negative emotions from time to time, the quicker we can do this and release them, then take a more philosophical approach, the better!

This is because the longer we manifest negative emotions and let them fester away within us, the more damage it's doing to us – that's both mentally and physically. The time frame within which this happens is referred to as our "refractory period" and the more we can limit this time the better.

We can do this by letting out negative emotion by safely releasing it (be that via a good cry or by shouting, having a rant, a grump etc.), then seeing it as just an "experience" and taking positive lessons from it. If we can see everything as an "experience" rather than attaching negative emotions to it, we can better maintain a positive focus, so that our experiences soon become memories without the emotional charge – and, ultimately, become wisdom.

The more of a positive focus we can keep and the more of an appreciation that everything (whether it was good, bad, or indifferent at the time) happens in order for us to learn something and move further along our path, the more positivity we'll attract back to us. This is based on the physical principle of "like attracts like", referred to as the "law of attraction".

To explore this further, in Chapters Four and Six there are plenty of resources and ideas to apply, particularly the tool of "reframing" – how to see things differently.

Positive thinking isn't ever as superficial as it might sound, either. It's never a case of "just be positive and everything will be fine", which people often mistake it for – the "Happy Clappy Club" label, so to speak. What it is in fact is conditioning yourself to make your predominant focus positive while still having a peripheral awareness of everything else.

Quite literally, we get what we focus on, and we see what we want to see, even if something is seemingly the same – for example, a brother and sister for example experiencing the same childhood event but each having very different memories of it simply because of the experience and emotion they each attach to it.

A simple metaphorical example is this image of a corner house below. Take a really good look at it.

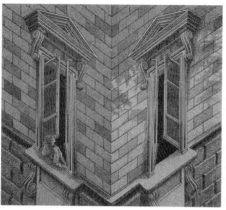

Photo by Bing Images, Artist Istvan Orosz

Depending on where you put your focus, either on the bottom half of the image or the top, you will see a different perspective. Use your palm to cover the upper part of the picture and look at it; then cover the lower part of the picture and look at it again.

Completely different, yes? But, obviously, it's always the same picture! The point being that you get the perspective you focus your attention on and decide to see. So, imagine: if one of these halves were positive and the other negative, which would you choose to focus on? Whichever one you choose, you will see – create – a different result than if you'd chosen the other.

3.   Always knowing and feeling your outcome at your deepest core level
- Why are you doing what you are doing?
- What is your ultimate purpose and intention?
- What do you want to achieve – what is your precise aim?
- Do you focus on what you want rather than what you don't want?
- Where do you spend most time putting your focus?
- Is this where you want it to be and are you focused on getting what you want?
- Do you waste too much time thinking and dwelling on the things you don't want and what "might" go wrong?
- Can you "feel" and really associate into what it is like when you have already achieved your outcome?

4.   Great behavioural and mental flexibility

- This is important for being able to successfully execute any goal (big or small); you need to be flexible enough in your thinking, if the first way you try to do something proves challenging or isn't working, to look at other options and ways instead.

- Behavioural and mental flexibility are vital to success. In my experience, with all-round flexibility anything is possible, as it helps put you in control of the situation. I've always got (eventually!) what I've wanted by being flexible and thinking outside the box.

- It's about seldom taking no for an answer, because there's usually another way to get over obstacles. There's always more than one way of doing something, no matter how unconventional it may seem – we just have to think about it.

- Life throws up plenty of challenges and obstacles, but if we have flexible thinking and behaviour, we can more often than not easily overcome these challenges.

- A key way of doing this is by using "lateral/ logical thinking". Start by asking yourself the question:

  – What is the main purpose, point and intention of something in the first place?
  – What's the bigger picture?

Once you get to this, ask yourself:

  – What are other examples of this – other ways/alternatives in which I could achieve the same thing?

Think about your challenges in the past, and whether, if you had had flexible thinking and behaviour at the time, could you have potentially got a different and more productive outcome? What factors can you change to make something seem better or more suitable?

- What else can you do about it?

In adopting this point, you'll naturally become a problem-solver, solutions-focused - focused on your outcome - as opposed to being focused on the problem. Be willing to change your thinking to get the results you seek. Change your own behaviour to adapt and "model/shadow" the right people where needed.

- Notice how people are responding to you.
- Do you need to change your tactics for better results?
- Notice small changes in others and the world around you so you can adapt your behaviour accordingly for the best outcomes.
- Notice changes and become observant of what works best and what you can change. Be aware of your own emotions and behaviour too – what could you do differently for an even better outcome?

5. Self-awareness – physically and psychologically

Be aware of your physical state. Have you ever seen someone standing slumped and looking down, and felt that they were oozing confidence? Probably not!

How we present ourselves physically tends to reflect what is going on psychologically, and vice versa. A confident look – standing or sitting upright, head and shoulders back – will help to generate a confident feel, and unsurprisingly this will help you to get better results and attract better things. It will in turn help to generate positive chemical releases in the brain, leading to calm and positive physical feelings. Even if you don't feel like smiling, do it – it will have a positive impact on your mood and the mood of others around you.

A startling example of the effects that physical bearing can have on us, on the results we attract and on our impact on others is the time when my partner and I went to deliver a "Well-Being in the Workplace" teacher training session in the context of health and enhanced professional performance at a primary school in the UK. In fact, I think we're both still feeling stunned by it . . .

On our arrival, we were greeted (if you can call it that) by one of the teachers. She plodded towards us dragging her feet, no smile, head towards the floor and shoulders slumped (this wasn't down to any disability – I'd checked beforehand). When we introduced ourselves and asked if she'd had a good day, in a very flat voice she answered, "Better now that's over."

This was before we had even met the rest of the group; when we did, much to our disbelief, many of them had the same general physical bearing and attitude. What's really interesting to note here is that the group also voiced verbally and projected through their attitudes and manner profuse negativity about everything we had to say (which was all very positive and proactive).

One teacher directly said to me (rudely, with offence intended) "I don't believe you can stop diabetes." I replied "Exactly, so *you* wouldn't stop it!

By this I meant that the teacher in question would never have been able to reverse diabetes if she were in that situation, because of her negative belief system that she couldn't. Quite simply, we become what we deep down, genuinely believe.

You can see clearly from this situation how the way we think, our mindset and deep belief system, physical bearing and manner and verbal communication (not just the words but things like tonality too) are all interlinked.

Fortunately, a small minority of the group, including the head teacher, had an upbeat physical manner: they sat up straight yet relaxed, smiled, looked alert and had a positive attitude. Interestingly, it was these people who seemed to get the most out of the session and through our feedback, follow-ups and talking extensively with some of these individuals, they continually experience great results in their professional and personal lives, despite having their challenges too!

So physiology is really important in terms of expressing how we feel, what we project to the world and the results we get. You only have to think of all the successful, happy people you know. Do you ever see them looking or behaving in the same way as most of the teachers described above?

Equally, being aware of our psychology is crucially important. Maintaining a "psychology of excellence" means remaining in control of our thoughts and emotions in order to control and maintain our internal and external state (our moods). This is important because although we know all too well that not everything in life is cheerful, and tragic things can happen, we still need to keep an overall positive outlook so that we can be resourceful and get the best outcome possible.

Psychologically speaking, get to know yourself. What are your triggers, your motivations, your deep values that make you tick or flip? What stories do you tell yourself and why – what's going on in your own internal reality? What do you really need to change? Knowing the answers to all these questions about yourself will assist you in moving forward and getting the things you want. Working through this book will help you to develop a keen self-awareness with a strong purpose.

6.   Take action and test things out

Very often people have some great plans, but do nothing about them – and consequently nothing happens.

It's important to just give things a go sometimes without overthinking it. None of us are perfect and get everything right first time, so never be afraid to just give things a try and have another go if they don't go according to plan. Research and trial and improvement is a wonderful thing – keep going! You know the saying: Rome wasn't built in a day – yet it was a great city once it was built, and it's certainly still standing!

7. Creating "change windows" – dare to be different!

It's only when we dare to be different from our usual selves with our usual fears, phobias and emotional baggage that real change can occur. So to do this we have to create what I refer to as "major moments". These are the times when we are presented with certain opportunities to actually make a different decision and act in a way we may have never done before, making a conscious transition to being a different personality, a new fearless one, excited about breaking boundaries . . . the new "you".

In doing this we then create what I call "change windows" – this is when we think, feel and behave differently, which essentially changes our entire neurology, sending different bio-chemical messages from brain to body and back again. This affects each and every cell throughout our entire nervous system, thus causing an enormous internal shift and creating, essentially, a new you, with new results.

The 30-Day Resilience-Builder Challenges

Start reconditioning and transitioning your mind and body for positive change today with the following 30-day warm-up resilience challenges. There's a challenge for every day over a month.

You can warm up to handling uncertainty by randomly choosing a number between 1 and 30 every day for a month and look at the list below to see what challenge it correlates to. Alternatively, you can work through the list from 1 to 30. Either way will give you new daily challenges.

These are all designed to help with self-challenge and breaking some common comfort zones to create positive change, and the point of each task is to complete it whether you like it or not, whether it seems pointless, silly or stupid . . . Do you have the flexibility to do it? Can you dare yourself to do something different? Can you lose your inhibitions, utilize humour and handle the uncertainty of the task and the response you'll get?

1. **Say "Hello, how are you?" and smile at five random people** who you don't know.

2. **Play a game with your friends of challenging one another** to integrate funny or random phrases into normal conversations. A good one to play with is the renowned funny British football

presenter, Chris Kamara's, expressions: "I don't know, Jeff" or "It's unbelievable, Jeff", or something like "razzamatazz", "fandabidozi", "cowabunga", "Willy Wonka" . . . Essentially, just have fun thinking of your own random funny phrases and getting them into everyday conversation. It's good harmless fun and acts as a little dare, starting to push your comfort zone. You'll undoubtedly make a few other people laugh too.

3. **Strike up an amiable conversation with a stranger** or acquaintance, or say something amusing or unusual, either in person or on email.

4. **Be assertive and honest – speak out** (albeit within reason!) Speak what is on your mind. Things that you might not otherwise have dared to say; perhaps something you don't really like or agree with! Go a day with no subjugation – push your boundaries.

I've had so many experiences where I've heard people complaining profusely among themselves or to me about something; yet when they have the chance to tell the person they really need to be telling to make a difference, the cat's suddenly got their tongue – nothing's said and nothing changes. So, if you want to change things, this is a great mini-challenge to start with.

5. **Wear something different from usual.**

    Something more colourful perhaps, smart, glamorous; casual if you're used to feeling "stiff" in your clothes all day – just something that's a positive change for you! Perhaps change your hair colour or style, change your make-up, go without make-up, grow a beard or moustache, conversely shave it off . . . You're no doubt getting the drift by now! In any case, note how different it makes you feel.

A client of mine initially came to me feeling demotivated, worthless and consequently spiralling into clinical depression, and although her full spectrum of challenges was complex, when I asked about how she spent most of her days from the moment she opened her eyes, I soon established that she paid no attention to herself and generally wore a T-shirt and leggings all day, every day. I suggested some changes – getting her hair restyled, changing its colour, getting up a little earlier to pay more attention to herself and dressing smarter – and she began to feel different. In time, she began acting differently and had a greater sense of pride and authority about her. Not surprisingly, this subconsciously also created a change in her behaviour and habits overall, and subsequently the responses she got from other people. It's the old classic – if you don't deep-down respect and value yourself enough to care, how can you expect others to?

6. **Make that phone call you've been putting off** or call family or a friend you've not spoken to for ages. Listen to those voice mails and plan to confront what you've otherwise been avoiding.

7. **Have a complete mobile phone and social media switch-off** for 24 hours – it's very liberating and certainly pushes boundaries!

8. **Travel alone** – In a context that you are unfamiliar with.

9. **Buy a copy of the *Big Issue*** (the street newspaper sold by homeless people or individuals at risk of homelessness, giving them the opportunity to earn a legitimate income) and have a conversation with the seller about how they came about to be selling it. And if you have the bottle to take it further, have a go at selling a few to give the seller a short break. If you don't have the *Big Issue* where you are, do something similar: buy a homeless person a drink or take them to lunch and listen to their story, or think of another act of kindness you can perform – for a stranger in need or perhaps a new colleague.

10. **Meditate.**

    See "Positively Utilize Music" in Chapter Four to point you in the right direction for guided meditation, and Chapter Six "Exploring Meditation" for further information about the subject.

11. **Look at yourself in the mirror and say to yourself aloud "I love who I am, and I enjoy what I do."** If you find you can't do this yet and don't like the answer as to why, say to yourself instead "I have the courage to change my life and I respect myself enough to do it."

12. **Use a different mode of transport.** Leave your car at home and take public transport, walk or cycle for a change. Or instigate learning to drive if you don't. If that's not feasible, just park further away from your destination to make yourself cover a greater distance. Just shake up your routine, even if – especially if! – it makes things a little less comfortable or easy for you.

13. **Do something different and fun midweek,** again to shake things up a little. Things like EscapeDrome™ experiences.

    EscapeDrome™ is excellent for fun and socializing as well as pushing boundaries and enhancing a range of skills through playing games.

    Essentially, it's a great licensed café bar with an enormous games library where you can hire tables to play all kinds of games, coupled with a fabulous escape room with 70-plus specialist EscapeDrome™ scenarios to have fun working through. This particular company also go in to businesses with this too, so maybe it's worth exploring for some fun, creativity, and even continued professional development in to your work. For more information on this specifically you can visit www.ludoraticafe.com

14. **Do something out of character or spontaneous that makes you feel a little uncomfortable** – but that isn't harmful in any way, neither for you nor anyone else. . . For me this might include leaving my handbag at home while I go for a coffee, because my bag contains provisions and everything that I consider necessary – but in reality I can probably manage without. For you this might be leaving your mobile at home for the day, not wearing your watch, going outright commando or not writing out a shopping list and changing where or how you do your food shopping.

15. **Visit somewhere you haven't been before**. It can be quite an adventure if you pick and travel in a certain direction and then simply follow the brown signs indicating tourist attractions to see where you end up, and what you end up doing. If you're feeling less adventurous, or that's not feasible, try going to a restaurant or coffee bar that's new to you. It's good to have a go at finding places without relying on your GPS satnav too.

16. **Let your hair down and loosen up**. Things like dancing around the house to loud music. Or go to a comedy evening - or even host your own!

17. **Randomly surprise someone with something nice**. From paying someone a compliment and showing your appreciation of them, to sending someone flowers or taking them to lunch for no apparent reason other than surprising them with a treat.

18. **Go and play on the rides in an adventure playground** – with or without kids! This is exceptionally liberating, fun and challenging at the same time, for many reasons!

19. **Go completely vegan for the day or have a sugar/gluten/caffeine/alcohol/smoking-free day**.

20. **Create a "life list"** (as opposed to calling it a "bucket list") – Language is important and this is about doing everything you want to do in life because you just want to do it, rather than waiting until you think time is short (remember we get what we focus on!). The life discovery model in Chapter Eight will help further with this.

21. **Say "No" to someone or something you usually do** that you don't really like doing but feel obliged or duty-bound to do.

22. **In a restaurant or café, order something totally different** from your usual choice.

23. **Find a way to surrender your control.** This might be letting your children have discretion over something you would usually decide, or handing control over to a colleague at work, letting your partner make all the decisions . . . however and whatever you must do to experience surrendering your usual level of control.

24. **Explore and start a new hobby or interest.**
This could be joining a health club; going to an interest group or society; starting a study course or cooking classes; personal development workshops; doing some voluntary work in your community; community policing; charity work; school reading schemes . . .

25. **Come up with some personal enjoyment time for yourself that you can commit to every week.** This can be as simple as giving yourself a couple of hours of personal time doing whatever floats your boat; as long as it's something that's special and indulgent for you.

26. **Ask for a pay rise or, if not relevant, ask for a discount!**

27. **Ask people what they like about you and what advice they would give you to enhance yourself or your life.** Then make a list of all the things you like about yourself and the things you're good at.

28. **Create something new!** This could be anything from an innovative invention to aid you in your daily life to an experimental recipe or writing a song; making your own clothes or children's toy; from designing a fun game to creating a new business.

29. **Take a random day off and do something different.** Head out to the coast, catch a movie at the cinema, go to an art gallery, book a hotel for the night, search the web for sites with discounted things to do . . . select something different and just go and do it.

30. **If someone asks how you're doing or how your day is going, give the response "Fabulous, thank you!"** and if they ask you why, say "I'm creating exciting positive change." Do this irrespective of any challenges you might be having that day – that's the resilience bit!

The things that you do may seem trivial; conversely, they may seem like a pretty big deal. It will depend on your specific anxieties, confidence level and fears. Either way, this list will bring its own challenges for you in some way, and will therefore help with building up resilience and confidence and stimulating a positive amount of adrenaline to help motivate and push you further, promoting the attributes needed to fully break your comfort zone. It's also worth considering how pushing your boundaries and participating in the 30-day challenges can positively shape your life in other ways . . . Imagine what could come of opening up to meeting new people, experiencing new things or behaving differently. In any case, it will create a different law of attraction for you (see Chapter Eight for more on this) – perhaps steering you in a direction you'd never previously considered, becoming good friends with someone you'd never have expected or being presented with prospects you've never before contemplated . . . who knows? But the more you push forward and get out there, the more you'll experience and the greater prospects you'll invite.

Fear Flipping

Have fun with creating your own list of resilience-builders, using the table below, by taking the things that are a comfort to you and giving yourself tasks that involve doing the opposite.

You can also list all the things that personally scare you and write down what the opposite of these would be. Then you can work out the specific task or challenge you need to do to overcome them. The more fun and creative you can make your fear-flipping tasks the better!

So, for example:

My Comfort Zone	My Fear/Anxiety	My Mission
Subjugating myself to others and following the crowd	Decision-making and leading – fear of being wrong and upsetting people	Create my own project – something that interests me – and practise asserting myself (see resilience-builder no. 4 above for ideas)
Remaining behind the scenes	Public Speaking	Get involved with larger groups of people – from meeting with more friends and family at once to new groups in the community, or business networking. Then start or lead the conversation within a small subgroup

It's important to remember that all irrational fear is in your head. Yours, mine – it's all subjective, hence why some techniques will work better for you than others.

All our fears are unique and different, born out of different experiences right from the moment of conception (some even before, if you're not afraid to go down that route) and often maintained through subconscious programming throughout life. For example, when we say to one another things like, "Be careful," "Safe journey," "Good luck," "Touch wood," "Have you had enough to eat?", we presuppose that something may well go wrong and so perpetuate our subconscious anxieties.

The later chapters of this book will help you to conquer such origins of fear once and for all, ultimately allowing you to meet with your life's goals and purpose. Because at the end of the day, the only thing holding any of us back is ourselves and how we process, manifest and deal with fear. Perhaps this sounds like a cliché, but it is nonetheless true!

> *"Do the thing you fear the most and the death of fear is certain."*
>
> Mark Twain

Summary

- When was the last time you did something that scared you, breaking your personal boundaries to push yourself forward in life? What was the fear that you overcame?
- Fear is never really the problem – it's what's behind it and how we think that's the issue. What one person can do, so can another – so what's the difference?
- There are seven key principles that will always ensure successful results:
  - Awareness that your internal reality is what creates your external reality.
  - Positive focus and limiting your refractory period.
  - Knowing and feeling your outcome at your deepest core level.
  - Having great behavioural and mental flexibility.
  - Physical and psychological self-awareness.
  - Taking action and testing things out.
  - Creating "change windows" – dare to be different.

The 30-day resilience-builder challenges will help to start reconditioning and transitioning your mind and body for change. You can create your own by "flipping your fear". All fears and limitations are individual and unique; however, there is something that can help everyone, meaning the only thing ever holding you back is you – a cliché, but 100 per cent true!

CHAPTER THREE

UNDERSTANDING FEAR AND WHY IT RESIDES IN ALL OF US

As we know, anything stopping us from stepping outside our comfort zone, doing everything we can and getting the results we want ultimately comes down to fear in one form or another, making awareness of this fear a fundamental key to success in anything. This chapter is therefore about really understanding how our brain and emotions work, and why we all have fears, whoever we are.

Fear resides in all of us, human or animal; we all instinctively respond to danger with natural defence mechanisms when we instinctively know we need to protect ourselves from harm.

In these scenarios the reptilian part of the brain, located in the brainstem and referred to as the instinctive alarm centre of the brain, provides us with an instant reflex action to protect us from harm before we have time to think and process what's happening.

For example, if a large object is zooming towards us we instinctively duck; when we're surprised by a loud noise we jump and react; or if we catch a glimpse of something slithery that might be poisonous we run! Our hearts start pounding and our palms begin to sweat— just two indications of the physical and emotional state we later experience and refer to as "fear" when we can start to process what has just happened.

So, one thing guaranteed in life is that we all have fears, and to be honest that's actually a good thing because we probably wouldn't be alive otherwise!

If we didn't fear falling to our death, we'd probably take some uncalculated risks when it comes to standing too close to the edge.

Similarly, if we didn't fear losing a loved one, we may never experience real love or be that concerned for their safety when we might need to be.

Here we're talking about instinctive fear, the fight-or-flight response that is inbuilt deep within us and which ultimately serves to protect us. The response that alerts our bodies to pump out a huge rush of adrenaline, allowing us to either run, hide or fight to protect ourselves. So, when we talk about confronting and overcoming fears, we're never referring to instinctive fear – that's yours to keep for life and save for emergencies – your instinct.

We also all experience natural fear, the kind of fear we need to push ourselves forward and grow. The kind of fear that helps us to build resilience. This should never be seen as a bad thing because we are living, evolving beings and such fear will always exist. It's simply conscientiousness and our minds telling us to focus – sometimes it can be confused with feeling anxious but actually this is just the physical feeling of our minds alerting us to focus.

However, it is useful to be aware whether this natural fear becomes unnatural, irrational and out of control, therefore holding us back rather than serving to push us forward.

So, all other fear . . .

Now that's an entirely different matter. And it comes in many different guises. Essentially, this is all irrational fear and serves no positive purpose; for example, it is perfectly natural to have a fear of losing a loved one BUT, fearing it to the extent of being worried sick about them every day, tracking their every move, feeling scared stiff and fearing our own loneliness – that's a problem!

The Only Two Emotions in the World

If we really delve deep, there are only two real emotions in the world: love and fear. All else is just a derivative of one of the two.

LOVE	FEAR
Joy	Frustration
Happiness	Anger
Laughter	Sadness
Fun	Hurt
Excitement	Guilt
Pleasure	Anxiety
Arousal	Pain
Contentment, satisfaction	Stress, worry

So, if we look at any undesirable or negative emotion, we can trace it back to a fear. Let's first take anxiety, a classic example. Being anxious about something, say, taking an exam, is likely to pertain ultimately to a fear of failure, of feeling not good enough, of not getting what we want. So whatever personal core reason we may have for being anxious about the exam specifically, it leads us back to fear.

Similarly, sadness at, say, a relationship break-up might ultimately pertain to a fear of being alone, of not having anyone with whom to share the good times or a fear of not being happy again or being good enough for anyone else.

So no matter how tenuous the link may seem, all the things that result in an undesirable or negative emotion can ultimately be traced back to fear.

A New Age Fear

Although fear has always existed and always will, in today's society it seems we are particularly besieged with a perpetual fear culture – what I call "New Age Fear".

"New Age Fear" because so many aspects of life, including people's personal lives, are widely exposed and subject to scrutiny, be this through social media or the general ease and speed of access to information via the internet. Essentially, this all gives rise to sensationalism, overwhelm, unrealistic expectations and getting drawn into the pressures of what is so often a false reality. The fast-paced, 24/7, technological world we live in today heightens what is anyway a rather fear-driven society.

Fear is increasingly apparent in everything from politics and social expectations to advertising and marketing: advertisers and social media culture encourage the fear of missing out, of not being glamorous/slim/rich/famous enough; politicians exploit the fear of losing money, of losing your job, of terrorism, of health threats, crime; the media manipulate thinking with fear . . . Everything seems to be so fear-driven; and, even worse, we're all growing more and more accustomed to it. Most of us are not consciously aware of the intense level of this existing cultural fear, but it is all constantly sinking in subconsciously and becoming the norm, despite the reality being something quite different.

This constant drip-feed of fear looping round and round in your brain brings some big challenges. It is mainly subconscious but nonetheless it results in those chemical changes that determine our moods and ultimately lead to the feeling of background anxiety that many people often experience without knowing why . . .

It's therefore important to be aware of this culture of subconscious fear and be able to tell the difference between a "real" embedded fear and fears that are just a product of our exposure to this culture. You can read more specifically about how this New Age Fear has manifested in our society at www.dr-em.co.uk in the articles section, "Where to draw the line in society!".

So, when does fear stop being rational and become a problem?

Well, if it's not a natural fear or an appropriate emotional response and you find it stops you from living your life, experiencing the world and getting the results you could otherwise get – then you could say, it's a problem! And here's why...

What Goes on Inside the Brain When We're Confronted with Fear?

When we experience a perceived threat through any one of our senses, it activates the amygdala, the area of the brain responsible for processing our emotional response. Responding to threat in fact involves many parts of the brain; however, the amygdala, an almond-shaped bundle of neurons buried deep in the brain, can be thought of as the catalyst in this process, the emotional epicentre.

The amygdala was first discovered to be the brain's "fear catalyst" when scientists noted that monkeys with damaged amygdalae were relatively tame and didn't show fear when confronted by snakes and other predators. Dozens of studies since have corroborated that damage to the amygdala coincides with abnormally low levels of a natural fear response – which is obviously very dangerous when it comes to having an instinctive response to danger.

This observation is not limited to other animals. In a study published in the journal *Current Biology*, researchers at the University of Iowa had worked with a woman with a very rare genetic condition called Urbach–Wiethe or lipoid proteinosis that destroyed her amygdala.

The study investigated the subject's response to frightening stimuli such as a haunted house, snakes, spiders and horror films, and asked her about traumatic experiences in her past, including situations that had endangered her life. They found that, as a result of not having a functioning amygdala, she is unable to experience fear.[1]

This highlights how significantly fear is linked to all emotion; hence when we can successfully control and work with our emotions (the basis of this whole book), we can overcome our unnecessary, irrational fears. When we perceive genuine, rational danger, the amygdala sends excitatory signals to other brain regions (the hypothalamus and pituitary gland) to release specific hormones that signal to our adrenal gland, located just above the kidneys, to release adrenaline and cortisol throughout the body. Adrenaline is responsible for the physical results we experience when we are scared, including a pounding heart, sweaty palms, increased respiration, shaking, a dry mouth and raised temperature. Cortisol is a potent immune-system suppressor and increases blood sugar; therefore, being repeatedly exposed to it can have very damaging effects.

When we experience a fear that is irrational, rather than an instinctive natural response, however, another part of the brain plays a central role. This is the hippocampus, which is responsible for storing and processing memories, and it gets involved because irrational fears tend to originate from memories, usually traumatic ones. The hippocampus then signals this fear to the amygdala, which does its job of triggering the emotional response to fear; which in turn triggers the chemical response of flooding our body with adrenaline and cortisol. And we experience the physical effects associated with fear, which are illustrated below.

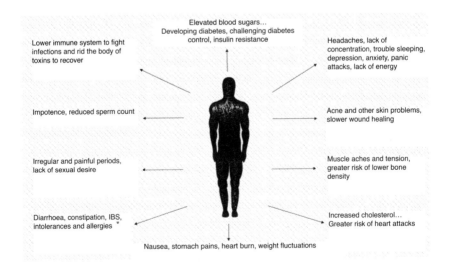

Elevated blood sugars...
Developing diabetes, challenging diabetes control, insulin resistance

Lower immune system to fight infections and rid the body of toxins to recover

Headaches, lack of concentration, trouble sleeping, depression, anxiety, panic attacks, lack of energy

Impotence, reduced sperm count

Acne and other skin problems, slower wound healing

Irregular and painful periods, lack of sexual desire

Muscle aches and tension, greater risk of lower bone density

Diarrhoea, constipation, IBS, intolerances and allergies

Increased cholesterol...
Greater risk of heart attacks

Nausea, stomach pains, heart burn, weight fluctuations

So, manifesting and holding on to irrational fears, phobias and any form of chronic stress or anxiety can eventually prove devastating to our health and well-being.

What do we need to do to start tackling this?

It all starts with what and how we think. This is because our thoughts affect our emotions and therefore our behaviours, physical health and the results we get in life.

The Cognitive Behavioural Cycle

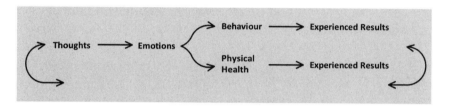

To understand this, think of public speaking, which is a very common fear that many people think of as a fate worse than death. In this situation:

- You imagine that something is going to go wrong – that you might forget your words, or say something wrong, causing people to laugh or poke fun. Then you think about how embarrassed, humiliated or uncomfortable you'd feel and how you'd want the ground to swallow you up.
- This then leads to the emotions of stress, anxiety and fear.
- Your body then begins to respond accordingly, as we've seen, by producing biochemicals in the brain that release adrenaline and cortisol to induce all the physical effects of panic.
- You then behave accordingly – you appear distracted, you DO forget your words, you struggle to speak clearly because your mouth is dry, have problems catching your breath and keeping hold of your train of thought . . .
- You experience the results of your talk not going well: maybe a lack of interest in your work and an absence of the opportunities you were hoping for.
- Next time you're in the same situation, the cycle begins again; you imagine that something is going to go wrong, exacerbated by your last experience . . .

We can, however, break this cycle and even change the biochemistry of the brain in the long term. These changes will form the basis of all our strategies to deal with whatever fears might present themselves in our lives from now on. However, even when we know our fears are irrational and we know the damage this can do to us – and how we can get help to do something about it – many of us still hold on to fear. Why is this?

Quite simply, this is often when fear is serving a greater purpose in one way or another, good or bad:

- The fear is ultimately creating pleasure and is deemed worth holding on to (a positive reason).
- We feel there is a far greater reason for suffering from the fear (a negative reason).

The Rush Effect – A Walk on the Wild Side

Fear isn't always a problem and certainly doesn't always require letting go of. In fact, in some instances people aren't even aware of just how much they utilize fear for positive results. This is something I refer to as the "Rush Effect" – the fun, pleasurable, exciting, energetic or euphoric effects of the mind and body's response to holding on to fear.

The term refers to the amazing feeling you get from the short blast of adrenaline driving you and then the exhilarating feeling of relief at having confronted or overcome a fear. This could be anything, from all the pent-up nerves of queueing up to ride a monster of a roller coaster and the brilliant feeling when you've done it to having performance anxiety or fears before public speaking or singing and then the high and rush of endorphins once you've done it, having utilized the anticipation to perform at your best.

This aspect of fear can be the driver for some people and can be the trigger that makes them great at what they do. Essentially, they are utilizing their fears and anxiety to feel good. This is a common phenomenon in people who take part in extreme sports, thrill-seeking activities or forms of sexual behaviour like BDSM. The commonality is that all these things induce fear, but the rush effect feelings of pleasure, joy and excitement override this, thus acting as a driver or trigger for people to push their comfort zones.

The rush effect can therefore act as a great alternative focus when you need to face your fears; rather than focusing on nerves, panic and the other intense negative feelings associated with fear and anxiety, focus instead on the amazing way you will feel afterwards – turn those nerves into anticipatory excitement and allow yourself to go for it with a redefined "fear" and renewed focus. There's more to help with this under "Reframing" and "Cleaning Up the What-Ifs" in Chapters Four and Six.

There is, however, another far more serious reason as to why we may hang on to fear, something I refer to as a "personal positive" and which is sometimes referred to more formally as a "secondary gain".

Personal Positives

This term refers to when, even though something is undesirable – maybe a fear or an illness – people still hang on to it because they get something else more positive out of having the fear or illness. This could be anything from getting a hug or special attention to feeling the reassurance of being looked after; perhaps someone might even gain celebrity status, a career or financial benefits from it.

Although these are, to a point, positive outcomes, hanging on to fear or illness is not desirable. So it's important, if this is something you recognize, to become more aware of it and address the root question: how else could you be getting what you need without having to go to those extremes?

Differentiating between Rush Effect and Personal Positive

Often, in my practice when seeing clients regarding any fear or limitation, at some point I'll ask "What do you LIKE about it?" and "How's it a problem exactly?" to help differentiate between the kinds of fear we experience, and to find what may be at the root of it.

Firstly, these questions tend to surprise people and help to start changing their thinking pattern; they can also help to identify a person's real thinking about their fear or anxiety, which is a step towards allowing them to feel differently by unravelling what else it can represent.

Where Does Fear Come From?

Assuming we're not talking about natural fear, which is normal and helps us to grow, or our instinctive reptilian response to protect ourselves, fear comes from one place . . .

It's all in your head!

Irrational fear isn't necessary, and most often isn't tangible. It's not even real at all; it is in your own mind and is just your personal perception of something and your personal manifestation of it. For example, three people may all be scared, fundamentally, of falling but one of them could manifest this as being afraid of heights, the second through being afraid of flying and the third through being afraid of riding big roller coasters. This is because we all process what might appear to be the same event, trauma or experience differently.

Our personal fears are born out of our individual experiences, beliefs and values, how we process our environment and what we interpret through our senses.

So we might learn a fear from our parents; from a religious upbringing or other very deep beliefs stemming from our childhood, or perhaps from experiences in which we have endured such hurt or trauma that we over-generalize these intense emotions by applying the negative emotions of that one bad experience to everything else akin to it thereafter. We then attach these feelings to one thing and subsequently develop a fear of that thing.

For example, say you are on a riding lesson but something startles your horse, causing you to fall off and have a bad accident. You over-generalize this experience by starting to think that "all" riding is dangerous. You then attach these feelings to horses and develop an intense fear of horses.

In my own case, I know my dislike of height originates from my grandma because I used to see her avoid them and say how much she didn't like them because they made her feel dizzy and nauseous. So from as early in my life as I can remember I have been learning to fear and avoid heights. And, although my sister and I in childhood experienced the same traumatic event, from it she developed an intense phobia of hospitals (which I talked about in the preface) whereas in my case I developed ill health; the physical effects of the fear I experienced weakened my immune system so much that it ultimately attacked my own body, resulting in Type 1 diabetes.

A client of mine feared public toilets; this fear originated from being raped in one when she was in her teens.

And my partner's once fear of reading aloud came from him having severe undiagnosed dyslexia as a child and being humiliated when forced to read aloud at school; this subsequently manifested a limiting belief that he was "thick", "stupid", "not academic" and so on.

So, you can clearly see a pattern of how our experiences can be so different and yet have a common effect in seriously impeding our lives.

Now we have looked at how fear works and resides within all of us, you can probably begin to see why there are so many ways available to us to confront and overcome our fears. There is, though, one thing that is universally true: it all starts with the mind; how we think and respond. So, once we positively change our thinking and approach to irrational fear, there really are no limits as to what we can achieve! The next step to consider is what we're prepared to do to overcome these fears.

"If you live in fear of the future because of what happened in the past, you'll end up losing sight of everything great that you have in the present."

Summary

- Anything that prevents us from stepping outside our comfort zone and breaking boundaries ultimately comes down to fear in one form or another.
- There are only two real emotions in the world: love and fear.
- Fear goes from the rational to being problematic when it's no longer a natural or appropriate emotional response and it prevents you from getting the results you could otherwise achieve.
- The brain produces specific neurochemicals in response to fear, which signal to the body to physically respond in certain ways. This is a problem when the stress caused by this is prolonged.
- Our thoughts biochemically affect our emotions, which in turn affect our physical health and behaviour and therefore the results we get in life.
- Irrational fears are born out of our individual experiences, perceptions, beliefs and values, making most fear not even real; hence we can all positively do something about it!

CHAPTER FOUR

BABY STEPS: THE ALL-IMPORTANT STEPS TO A FIRM FOUNDATION

Although it's quite feasible for some of us to dive straight in when it comes to facing our fears, a good warm-up often makes for a better performance and result. In this case, it all starts with good mental preparation. So, here are tips and tricks that you can practise and utilize when it counts.

Your Essential Toolkit

Knowing how to get into the zone and learning different breathing patterns are two of the most simple but effective techniques – they will both change your state in an instant.

Getting in the Zone

This technique is used widely by top sports professionals and the special forces. It is very simple but very effective. It helps to focus your attention in the right way, relax, remain stress-free and successfully go about your task. When practised and applied properly, in this state the brain is unable to access negative emotion – fear being the principal negative emotion here.

- Focus on a spot in front of you, just above eye level.
- Notice everything about this spot – size, shape, colour, purpose.
- While still heavily focused on the spot, expand your vision 180 degrees either side of you to notice what is in your peripheral vision – at the same time as still focusing on the spot above eye level.

Peripheral vision technique, breathing, and relaxation state

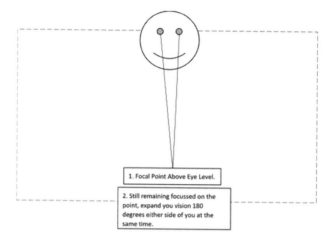

- Take a deep breath in through your nose (count to five) and exhale through your mouth (count to five). Visualize and feel the sensations of your breath running freely like water through your entire body, oxygenating every cell with life-force energy.
- Repeat to yourself, "Invigorated and transformed."
- Then visualize a beam of light and energy travelling up through the floor and throughout your body; as the light shines, you feel positively energized, calm and relaxed.

Breathing Techniques

Breathing is, obviously, something we do every day; but generally speaking we do it on autopilot and don't pay much if any attention to it – until it becomes compromised in some way: through panic attacks, various health conditions, anxiety, anger or, of course, fear. However, by paying positive attention to our breathing we can significantly improve our general health as well as our emotional and physical state.

Respiration occurs within our body's cells. This is the process whereby nutrient fuel is burned with oxygen to release energy; if our oxygen supply is restricted this process becomes unbalanced and our cells (and thus our organs) are unable to function optimally. Hence the brain being starved of oxygen can lead to brain damage or death. Conversely, if we take time out to focus on our breathing, we can increase our energy and optimize cell function, allowing for maximum health and a state of calm and well-being.

Practising the following breathing techniques regularly can therefore be very beneficial. They can also be practised "on the spot" in times of stress or panic, to help bring the breathing back to normal. If you become dizzy at any point while doing any of these techniques, stop and let your breathing regulate, take a few minutes to sit still, then sip a drink of water.

To bring the breathing back under control, take a deep breath in through your nose (count to four) and exhale through your mouth (count to four). It can help to imagine drawing a circle or clock in your mind, starting at 12 and drawing breath at 3, 6, 9 and back to 12.

Try the following for life-giving, calming energy:

Ocean Breath

Inhale deeply through your nose and exhale through your mouth as if you are fogging a mirror; however, do this with your mouth only slightly open. Make this cycle rhythmic and continuous like the rolling sound of the ocean. Repeat for five minutes.

Now take three deep breaths and change to

Fire Breath

Inhale and exhale rapidly through your nose only as if you are constantly sniffing, using your abdomen as a "pump". Repeat for five minutes.

Now relax, notice the sensations throughout your body and stretch – you may notice that you are feeling more energized, calm and relaxed. You may even notice tingling sensations throughout your body; this is perfectly normal.

Changing How You Think

When you begin to change the way you think about things, the things you think about begin to change – then you can expect to experience different results!

I shared with you earlier my once-overwhelming phobia of heights, which I eventually overcame by having to confront it because I unexpectedly had to deliver a training session on the top floor of a skyscraper hotel. I openly admit, though, that had this not been for an important organization, with a stipulation that only I could deliver the session, and had everyone not already been there waiting for me, I would have likely sent somebody else to replace me!

So, what made the difference in my mind that really made me confront this fear?

Well, quite simply, it was thinking differently from how I had been thinking previously.

The only reason any of us do anything is because of our values, what's important to us; this gives us the motivation to act. In my case, a sense of duty and professional diligence is extremely important to me and on this occasion I wasn't just responsible for myself, there was a lot riding on the decision I made. In other words, it wouldn't just have been me I was letting down; and there would have been other, far-reaching consequences too.

This meant that the once-unthinkable suddenly became something I was ready to confront for the greater good. I just did it, simply because my thinking had changed: everything else remained the same.

Similarly, if I saw someone about to jump off a high-rise building, I wouldn't think twice about rushing up there to help talk them down.

Ultimately this boils down to having a bigger distraction, focus and purpose than just me and my nerves.

So, changing how we think is key to changing how we feel, and therefore it is how we can suddenly become capable of different behaviour. I have discussed already some of the weird and wonderful ways to do this, but it all starts with adopting a different mindset and way of thinking.

Remember one of the three solutions to overcoming certain fear and breaking out of our comfort zone is putting ourselves in the space whereby we have no choice but to simply do the things that scare us; and getting to this is about taking small steps and building up a resilience to make mastering any ultimate fears a pleasant walk in the park – thus focusing more on the rush effect.

Reframing

This simply means giving something a different frame, or having a different take on your thinking about something. Essentially, reframing is changing how we look at something and seeing it in a more positive and constructive context. Below is a classic example.

In my practice I saw a lady who had severe clinical depression and was also seriously afraid of death. So (much to her surprise) the first thing I said to her was, "Excellent! At least we know you're not at risk of suicide; I'd say that's a pretty useful phobia to have in this context!" This instantly established a smile, as well as an altered way of thinking about her challenges – being afraid of death but simultaneously afraid of living – and she soon experienced the two cancelling each other out. The end result – a very happy and well individual, embracing life as she currently knows it.

Cleaning Up the 'What-If's'

Imagine a time when you might have had a doubt over something that has led to you feeling besieged by a tonne of other negative thoughts, soon followed by that exceptionally uncomfortable feeling of overwhelm; it has then got so out of hand that it has blocked you even more from doing whatever you were fearful or anxious about in the first place – and ultimately has stopped you from doing or achieving what you wanted to.

This experience is horrible. But it's something most of us can relate to! There's one simple way to overcome it and that's to seriously practise, until it becomes second nature, what I call "cleaning up the what-ifs": seriously cleaning up that distracting conscious clutter. Here's how:

Write down or say out loud your "what if" fears; for example:

- What if I'm not good enough?
- What if I fail?
- What if I make a fool of myself and people laugh, and then I feel embarrassed/humiliated?
- What if I don't have the finances?
- What if people will think I'm different, stupid, mad . . .

It doesn't matter what your what-ifs are or how big or small; they're important to you and they're blocking your energy to be where you want to be in life. Just note them all down and also note any significant negative emotion behind them – these might include embarrassment, humiliation, sadness, disappointment, . . .

Then ask yourself:

- "What's the worst thing that can happen if . . .?" Does it really matter in the grand scheme of life?
- "When was the first time I ever felt that particular negative emotion, and what significant event can I link it to?" For example, were you ever embarrassed or humiliated at school for getting something wrong? Consider anything, no matter how seemingly small or insignificant.

In relation to point one, you'll have likely surmised that whatever it is it won't kill you – or it's exceptionally unlikely to! Otherwise you're probably dealing with rational fear and need to explore "the law of attraction" and "Quantum reality", to be found in Chapter Eight.

In relation to point two, for now just keep the answer in mind. It will help to run through the RACE™ technique in Chapter Six so you can remove any associated root fears ultimately causing the what-ifs.

Back to point one . . .

Begin cleaning up these what-ifs by rationally questioning what else they might mean and by looking at the converse – the opposite that starts to emerge when you flip your thinking, like:

- What if you ARE good enough and you ARE a resounding success?
- What if there's no such thing as failure if you see everything as constructive feedback to push you further forward and you're out there having a go?
- What's embarrassing about going for what you want, believing in yourself and having the strength to put yourself out there?
- What if you just don't have the finances YET; you are resourceful, and you are simply waiting for the right investor or opportunity to present itself, which will serve you better in the end?
- What if the negative or judgemental opinions of others are just their own projections and limitations, making it more about them than you?
- What if there are plenty of people to help and support you in whatever way you need if you are ready to look, and really believe in what you want? Chapters Six to Eight will help further with this.

When you work on your what-ifs you'll soon start to notice your worried thought patterns lift, as with any attached negative energy associated with the overwhelm experience described earlier. As you'll learn progressing through the following chapters, as your thinking patterns and belief system change, you will equally lose stored negative energy, which has a significant bearing on how everything else in your life will start to positively change too – something that is very exciting.

Although you can positively change your what-ifs around quickly to transform a situation, you can also look at these more extensively to create more positive solutions too. This directs your focus from worrying to proactively looking at the opportunities presented and the positive version of what something might mean. For example:

- Instead of accepting that you're not good enough in a certain area, think of what would happen if you underwent some new or extra training – what else do you need to learn or do, and where could this lead you?
- Could it make sense for you to enlist the help of others if the above isn't appropriate? Such an option might create the extra time for you to do a far better job on something else. It may even provide you with a much-needed break to increase overall productivity!
- Instead of thinking no one will help you financially, try changing it to "The right person will help". Although getting finance and investment is often a challenging process, it's usually not the case that no one is interested or it's unattainable; rather it tends to be because the right people/organization haven't come along for you, the timing isn't right or there's something else that you need to learn or do before the right opportunity can present itself. It's therefore worth exploring whether you have any deep, often unconscious, limiting beliefs, such as "I don't really deserve it" or "I'm not really worthy and capable of getting investment."

So rather than thinking and accepting that you can't get investment, think instead about what you need to look at to achieve it. Chapters Six to Eight will help with this self-awareness and help reveal any personal blockages – a powerful enlightening process that can make all the difference.

- You can change the context in which you think about things like embarrassment too. For example, isn't it more embarrassing to give up on something you've been working for than to wholeheartedly give it everything you have with courage and determination?

Habitual Thinking and Changing Those Habits

If you've manifested a fear for a long time then you may well have got used thinking about it in a habitual way – and as we know, thoughts affect our emotions and our emotions govern our behaviour. Also, because other people are familiar with us displaying a certain fear, phobia or behaviour and therefore expect a certain reaction, we sometimes feel almost obliged to hang on to it or draw out an emotion. However, despite this, with a little work we can change our state very quickly. Ways to work on looking at things differently include:

- Looking at what else your fear or limitation can mean – What can you positively learn from it, what life lessons can this teach you, what positive resources do you need to adopt from this experience?
- Looking at the positive alternative meaning of words. If you notice yourself using language that casts doubt on your belief that you can do something, change disempowering fear words to empowering positive words. Use The Word Exchange table below as a guide.

THE WORD EXCHANGE

Negi-tude Words	Replacement Power Words
Nerves	Anticipation and excitement
Problems	Challenges and opportunity
I can't	I can if . . .
It's not my fault	Where's my responsibility?
I'm anxious	I'm aware and conscientious
I'm discontent	I'm finding focus and purpose
Disaster	Opportunity/learnings
Life's a struggle	Life's an adventure
I hope	I know, I trust . . .
If only I'd . . .	I can learn and know next time . . .
I'm stuck	I'm resourceful
It's awful	I learn from it or focus on helping
There's nothing I can do	I'm creative
I'm old and getting past it	I have great, invaluable experience
I resent so much	I forgive by appreciating the "why"
I'm empty	I can be fulfilled
I'm lonely	I'm open and connected
It costs too much	It's an investment and has value
I need to control	I can trust and let go
At least . . .	It's great that . . .

- By changing the context of your fear, could you make it positive? For example, say you were petrified of clowns. Could you confront this by BEING the clown at a charity event? Is it possible to fear yourself? Can you make things humorous, enjoy the fun and simultaneously raise money?

The Art of Self-Questioning

Self-questioning can really help to get things into perspective when you're feeling fearful or out of your comfort zone in any context. In some cases, it can even dissolve the problem altogether by allowing you to get to the heart of the matter. You do this by looking beyond the immediate problem and using a process of deduction (gradually breaking things down). This then allows you to see how some things aren't really a problem at all, subsequently encouraging you to confront and test your challenges.

Questions for Yourself

- Does it really matter right now? Is it really that important in the grand scheme of life? Is this stress/anxiety/fear worth sacrificing my health for?
- If I were to die tomorrow, would there have been any point in being so fearful and wasting time over it?
- Would it matter or make any difference if I did or didn't stress and feel fearful about it at present?
- What is fear really going to achieve, if something is going to happen anyway? What's the best, most productive action I can take to get the best possible outcome given the situation?
- Is my focus in the right place? What is my main purpose and intention in doing this thing – the big picture? Is stressing and being fearful helping me to create the right focus? Remember the corner house from Chapter Two and how we see what we focus on, even if we're aware of other things.
- How, specifically, is something a problem? What is preventing me from reaching a solution and moving forward?
- Am I being as resourceful as I could be? What can I do about it? What

resources do I have available to me? What can I be grateful for and show gratitude for?

- Is fear just a waste of life? What is it I like so much about it? Could this be a good thing? Could I enjoy this aspect in another more productive, healthier way?

Change Your Focus

Give your mind positive messages or mantras, rather than (as a lot of people do) an extensive range of profanities coupled with "I can't do it!"

Have a go instead at repeating something positive or fun, or just a distracting bit of nonsense:

- "Have some fun and get it done . . . A do it, A do it NOW . . .! Ding, Ding".
- "He who dares wins" – Del Boy, a character from much-loved British sitcom *Only Fools and Horses*.
- "Screw it, just do it" (evoked before but it is very useful!) – Richard Branson, British entrepreneur.
- "It's unbelievable, Jeff" – Chris Kamara, British sports presenter.

Be creative – try them in funny voices and accents too. Use other famous quotes that you like or you come across.

Create an Outcome

Give yourself a reward, something to look forward to – or, if it works better for you to think of it this way, you can't have a certain something unless you do "x".

Make Yourself Accountable

Tell someone what you're going to do so you feel more pressure to go through with it and it's not as easy to bottle out of. This might be, for example, doing something for charity, your boss or your friends; or simply going public with something utilizing social media.

This is a great tactic to "put yourself in the space", making it challenging to go back on your word and leaving you little choice but to just do it!

Model Someone and Pretend

If we pretend and practise something for long enough, we become it! With this in mind, pretend to be someone who you deem to be confident, fearless, humorous – whatever features you would like more of for yourself. Adopt all their positive attributes, including their physical manner – how they look and hold themselves – their values and their attitude to things – just as if you are acting or doing an impression of them.

Can you imagine modelling Oprah Winfrey's courageous attitude, energy, drive and determination for positive change?

Ray Kroc's unshakable belief system (He was the hugely successful American businessman, known for his revolutionary ideas, who made McDonald's the phenomenal global success it is today). For inspiration, watch the 2016 film about Kroc and McDonald's, *The Founder.*

Or you could choose to model someone you know personally and who you admire. Even poke fun in a humorous way if it helps get you into the right state.

If modelling someone seems a bit daunting, try just doing an impression of an individual, either real or a character from a TV show, or film, or anywhere else you admire. Even just doing a brief, throwaway impression involves making neurological shifts as you release the chemicals to cause the physical changes that enable you to impersonate the other person. This is enough to make a change in your mood and behaviour, or maybe give you that extra push you need to achieve something.

Positively Utilize Music

Listen to music that really builds you up and evokes positive strong emotions in you – if you want to feel unbeatable, for example, try the soundtrack from *Rocky.* A bit of a cliché, maybe, but there's a reason why many people use it for training and exercise! Music can really set a mood and change your state, acting as a subconscious trigger to motivate you in a particular way. Music can even alter your brainwaves and therefore your mental state. EEG studies conducted at Duke University in North Carolina have concluded that binaural beats have the potential to affect mood and performance.[2]

Binaural beats (two marginally different frequency levels of the same sound sent to each ear through headphones) balance the right and left hemisphere of the brain by matching the overall sound frequency with brainwaves and heartbeats measured when people are in certain optimal states. So music can be specifically designed to slow down brainwaves, taking us into the ideal states of consciousness for relaxation, goal focus, performance enhancement, learning, meditation, healing, sleep and behaviour-changing.

In addition, research from Harvard Medical School, National Institutes of Health and *Psychology Today* agrees that binaural beats, brainwave entrainment (altering brainwaves for relaxation or focus), guided meditation and positive subliminal messaging (positive suggestions embedded in the mind) have a real and profound impact and benefits[3]. They are well worth investigating.

You will be able to find the right music for you, along with guided meditation audios, at www.brainsync.com.

Alternatively, you can also search online for alpha, theta or delta wave/binaural beat music.

Change Your Environment

Changing your environment can very easily change the way you think in two important respects:

- By using all your senses to visualize and imagine you are somewhere else – a safe, fun, happy place. This will automatically trigger positive emotions and so alter your thinking and therefore how you feel and subsequently act. There is more on this technique (which I refer to as using a "resource anchor") later on.
- Make sure the people in your environment are of a positive and encouraging nature because as negativity breeds, so does fear. So if you are around people who also share your phobias, fears or lack of confidence about certain things, it will only exacerbate how you feel. However, if you're surrounded by very positive, proactive people, it will encourage you to positively get on with things and cast a different perspective as positivity also breeds! An easy way to understand this is to imagine two agoraphobics living together – how often do you think they'd go out? Conversely, if a person with agoraphobia lived with a positive and proactive person, then the chances are this person would encourage the other to venture out more.

Create a Strong Resource Anchor – A Positivity Trigger

An anchor or trigger is a particular physical stimulus (an object, visual, sound, taste, smell or action) that automatically stimulates a certain response in how we think and feel; it evokes certain emotions, memories and associations, causing us to respond accordingly. This then naturally affects our state of mind – either positively or negatively.

A common example is when a certain song (the stimulus) comes on the radio and triggers us to automatically feel happy, energized, pensive or even sad because deep in our mind we link it to a specific stand-out experience where the song had particular relevance. For example, a song that got played when you were younger might evoke emotions of fun. Equally a song that was played at a family member's funeral might evoke sombre feelings.

We can therefore create our own positive anchors to evoke at any time to induce any feelings we like, usually calm and positive ones. So anchoring can be used to help change our state of mind – and of course, the results we get in many contexts.

- First, close your eyes and take some long, deep breaths (inhale through your nose and exhale through your mouth) to slow down your breathing. As you relax and your heart rate slows, feel the oxygen flowing easily throughout your entire body as you begin to relax deeper and deeper, allowing conscious clutter to float out of your mind.
- Now remember a time when you were really relaxed, calm, confident, content and happy – perhaps on a lovely holiday, in a spa, the garden or whatever works for you. See that time through your own eyes as if it were happening right now:
  - *See* the things you saw.
  - *Hear* what you *heard.*
  - Really *feel* the *feelings* of being calm, relaxed, and confident.
  - *Smell* any apparent *scents* of your surroundings – especially if it's the fresh sea air, grass, sunscreen, flowers, food and so on.
  - *Conjure* any *tastes* you may have had.
- Use all your senses in this way to experience that time again, as if it were happening right now.
- Once you are engrossed in this experience and totally reliving it, when it is at its most intense point, snap your thumb and first finger together sharply.

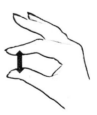

- As the imagined experience starts to fade, release your fingers and open your eyes.

You have just created a positive, calm anchor (a positive trigger) that you can apply whenever you are stressed to automatically induce those positive feelings. All you have to do to activate this is snap the same fingers together and this physical action will automatically trigger those same positive feelings connected to the experience you initially linked to it.

If other triggers work better for you, such as scents or music, you could spray or rub a particular scent onto a piece of cloth or a handkerchief you can keep with you in a pocket. You can use it to stimulate the positive feelings whenever needed.

Sometimes I wear a particular perfume because it reminds me of a happy memory in a favourite place of mine; it triggers feelings of being positive, calm and happy. For a similar effect, you could download a certain piece of music to your phone so you can easily access it to quickly change your state.

You can also use what I call a "gratitude rock" as your positive anchor. Carry with you any stone – a stone from the ground, your garden, a precious stone, a gemstone; whatever feels significant to you – and every time you touch it, think of something positive and joyful that you are grateful for in your life. It can be something big or small, as long as it means something to you. This will act to enhance positive focus too.

Visualization

Visualization is an incredibly powerful technique, and when properly understood and applied it has fantastic results. As the mind generally thinks in pictures and uses all our senses to create memory, using strong imagery can engrave positive messages deep into our neurology and effect physical changes.

Through research using PET scan technology, we know that through the action of powerful neurotransmitters, the same parts of the brain are activated whether subjects are vividly imagining something or experiencing it in reality; the nerve-firing and chemical release are so similar as to allow the mind to influence the body in the same way.

In other words, the part of the mind responsible for running and maintaining our body 24/7 on autopilot is unable to recognize the difference between what is real and what is not real.

If you've ever had a very realistic, vivid dream and woken up crying, laughing, or stimulated, disturbed or unsettled by it, then you have experienced this. Although it was "just a dream", it stimulated a physical response because your body believed it to be real and responded accordingly. You may even have had to question whether or not the event in your dream really happened!

We can widely use visualization as a powerful tool when it comes to being outside our comfort zone in many contexts. Visualization can assist in the healing process and activate simple physical changes, such as temperature control, lifting our mood and achieving goals. This is because if we visualize something with enough detail and clarity, our minds will instruct our bodies to physically respond accordingly and make the necessary changes.

One particular case, documented in 1971 by Dr O. Carl Simonton,[4] a radiologist at the University of Texas, involved a 61-year-old man who had been diagnosed with throat cancer. The cancer was very far progressed; the man could hardly swallow and his weight had dropped to 98 pounds. His prognosis was very poor: doctors gave him only a 5 per cent chance of survival after treatment and strongly anticipated that he wouldn't respond well to treatment, as he was already so weak.

Dr Simonton was curious as to whether he could find a psychological approach using visualization. He suggested that the patient visualize his immune system attacking the cancer, sweeping the cancer cells from his body and replacing them with healthy ones. The patient then went away and applied this visualization at regular intervals throughout the day. Shortly thereafter, the tumour began to shrink, and the patient's response to radiation was almost free of side-effects. Two months later, the tumour had completely disappeared!

This is a case of a successful recovery utilizing the power of the mind and shows that where a positive mindset and belief system are present, anything is possible. This same patient went on to use visualization to get his arthritis to disappear and remained free of this condition and the cancer during the six-year follow-up period, after which he resumed a regular healthy life. Imagine the limitations on his life if he had let fear of exploring the unconventional get in the way of his recovery.

In my professional practice we have seen clients make amazing recoveries from all kinds of manifested fears as a result of using the visualization techniques described in this book.

Norman Cousins (known for his immense personal and professional success in the field of healing and psychology) states: "The human mind converts ideas and expectations into biochemical realities"[5] and, of course, it is this that makes all the difference in the results we experience. This may be in any context applied to fear, either psychologically, physically through ill health as discussed in Chapter Three – by way of the neurochemicals and toxins generated from fear and chronic stress that compromise the immune system – or practically speaking by way of limiting the results we experience in life.

Chapter Six features more visualization techniques to release deeper fears and phobias that work with root causes on a more intense level than the techniques discussed in this chapter. Your essential toolkit techniques are rather designed for quick, simple use to apply when needed. However, here is a simple visualization technique to help with performance anxieties and fear that you can easily implement when needed.

In your mind, fly into the future, just after the specific event you are feeling anxious or nervous about. Clearly visualize a big success, something that signifies you've done a good job and achieved the outcome you want.

Make sure you really get into this. See what you can see through your own eyes as if you were experiencing it right now. Hear the things you can hear. What are people saying? What are you saying to yourself or others? Finally, really feel all the positive emotions you can feel – all those great, warm and satisfying feelings. Use all your senses, even any appropriate tastes and scents that are present. Really go for it – no holding back on your success!

Now lock this in your mind. Seal it in tight, so it stays right there. Stick it down, lock it in and throw away the key!

Now come back to the present and keep focused on that successful outcome awaiting you. Remember: what you focus on, you attract; so keep it positive. Keep seeing the outcome you want, and take all the practical, realistic actions necessary to achieve it. It's important to acknowledge and remember that as well as visualizing something, we must still take the necessary practical steps to achieve it.

For example, when I was first invited to teach a training course by myself in the United Arab Emirates, I visualized it in advance as being a great success. However, I still had to do all the preparation necessary to make this happen, such as making my projector slides, creating excellent course content and so forth. By visualizing success, though, I knew my intended outcome, and this ensured that any anxiety I felt was expressed as positive energy, allowing me to perform at my best rather than forgetting my words or messing up the delivery of the excellent training sessions I had planned for my clients.

In a nutshell: strongly visualize what success after the event will look and feel like and perform the necessary steps to ensure success. If you do that, then you will successfully transform any anxiety you are feeling into positive energy to ensure successful results.

Change Your Internal Representation

Have a go at transforming the feeling of nerves and anxiety into a feeling of excitement.

See fear as merely a challenge to be overcome and a character-building test of your determination to overcome certain issues in life.

Bring it on and give fear the finger – because you can.

Remember that unless natural fear is there to protect you, it's serving no positive purpose. It's holding you back and, frankly, it's winning. And you deserve better than that!

In applying all these resources and utilizing them when needed, you will soon develop your very own toolkit to be able to do the best mental preparation for anything you fear or are simply feeling anxious or apprehensive about.However, it's also important to remember that anxiety can be helpful and a manifestation of our unconscious mind alerting us to focus. You have all the essential tools, so now positively focus and channel your energy. You really can be unstoppable!

Considering a Comparison Frame for a Problem Blowout

Often when we think something is a much bigger problem or issue than it actually is, it creates an internal reality that is often very different to the external reality. In this situation, the simple principle of creating a comparison frame can really help put things into perspective and get you thinking differently and therefore responding more positively.

As the old saying has it, "There is always someone else worse off." Associating into, or really feeling, the reality of this will help you to appreciate what you do have and know that you can handle it and you do have the resourcefulness to deal with it – you'll always cope!

After terrible events such as the suicide bombing in Manchester in the UK, or 9/11 in New York, or in any disasters anywhere for that matter, we see what happens when people change their focus from themselves to helping and caring for others. Often in such circumstances their own challenges pale into insignificance, seeming unimportant in comparison.

This is a fairly extreme kind of scenario; but the point is that sometimes certain events will make something else suddenly seem far less important to you. Such as when children are around, or a personal matter takes over from work worries.

Often in my practice I work with clients on matters from clinical depression to chronic conditions and illnesses like cancer; it certainly keeps life in perspective.

When you do feel that something is a problem, or it's causing you anxiety, it's important to avoid getting sucked into it or giving it energy, as this only enables it to "grow" and seem more significant than it perhaps is. You'll also see in Chapter Eight why giving anything negative more focus and energy attracts even more of it. Just by taking ourselves out of the environment in which a problem exists, we can think differently about it, put things into perspective and often find a solution.

"Forget Everything and Run or Face Everything and Rise."

Zig Ziglar

Summary

- Methods using peripheral vision and specific breathing techniques are great instant ways to help focus and get in the zone in the moment, for better performance when it really matters.
- When we change the way we think about things, the things we think about change – then we can expect to experience different results!
- Being aware of and cleaning up our "what-ifs" can completely flip fear.
- There are many ways to "reframe" situations, allowing us to think and feel positively different.
- You have the resourcefulness to handle whatever is thrown your way. Therefore, you will always handle it, and you will always cope – with the right mindset.

CHAPTER FIVE

MINDSET MASTERY

Mindset is everything. It determines our character, the paths we choose and the results we get in life. By adopting the concepts and suggestions in this chapter, the resources throughout this book and your own great strengths you'll always ensure an indestructible mindset fit for maximum success, whatever challenges life may throw at you.

An incredible example of this and some of the key issues discussed in this chapter is Tommy Wiseau, producer, director, star and financier of the 2003 film *The Room*, which is widely described as "the worst film ever made". However, here's the point: Wiseau was so set on being a famous actor that, despite every challenge he encountered (namely that he wasn't great at it!), every critic and doubter, his sheer mindset and belief system still ensured that he succeeded in achieving fame and fortune: *The Room*, "the worst film ever made", has paradoxically had a successful and acclaimed film made about it, 2007's *The Disaster Artist*. "Seemingly", because it was Wiseau's law of attraction, his determined and unshakable positive belief in himself, that determined where his focus and energy went, therefore determining the positive energy he attracted back to him, despite the odds. Wiseau knew what he wanted, and he got it – so good, bad or indifferent, he achieved the fame he wanted on the big screen!

You may like to look online for an interview with Seth Rogen, star of *The Disaster Artist*, on the U.S. TV show *Late Night With Seth Meyers*, in which he talks about the film. The way he talks about Tommy's character will reinforce exactly why the points you read in this chapter can seriously make all the difference!

The Components of an Indestructible Mindset

If you know that you are always in control of your own mind and body, you'll also know that you are equally in control of the results you get, through what we choose to accept, think and act upon.

An important question here is, if you're not in control of your own mind, who is? If we take personal responsibility for everything we do, we will always be empowered to change things to how we want them. But if we look for external reasons as to why we haven't got the results we want, we immediately lose any power to take control and positively change things.

Remember: Reasons equate to being a victim, self-responsibility equates to change and results.

While there are always external factors beyond our control, we can always take charge of our own mind and control how we think and what we do; which will help to bring the external under control in line with our core deep-seated beliefs (see below). Reading this book is great proof that you can take control to make positive changes in your life – internally and externally. Keep going and it will come!

Maintaining Excellence

By this I mean controlling what's going on inside in order to control the way we externally look, behave and respond, thus the results we ultimately get.

This also includes the messages we give off to others around us. If we stay conscious of positively maintaining our inner thought process to maintain an inner resourceful state, despite being tired, stressed, or whatever else we are dealing with, we will always be able to manage things better and get the best results possible. The most successful people in the world – be they presidents, emergency service personnel or Olympic medallists – maintain a state of excellence, psychologically and therefore physically, which allows them to achieve distinction in what they do.

Lizzy Yarnold, the British 2018 Winter Olympics skeleton competitor, is a great example. Just before her race she had been suffering from a bad chest infection; she was struggling to breathe and partake in practice runs, and it was looking unlikely that she would be able to race. However, with great courage and motivation she took the decision to go out and give it her all anyway. And she won gold!

Never Be Afraid of Change

We can all change as much as we want to change – and when we do, we'll also notice the world around us changing, too. Without change, we can't expect to get different results. Positive change is fundamental to life and moving forward. Albert Einstein summed this up perfectly: "The definition of insanity is doing the same thing repeatedly and expecting different results."

Change is one of our greatest fears. It's not always comfortable and it often involves uncertainty (certainty being a psychological human need); hence it's understandable that we can easily feel out of our comfort zone when it comes to change. However, it is also what pushes us forward. If we change, everything around us changes too, including the results we get. And in any case, if something doesn't produce the results we like, we can work on changing it again until we do get what we want.

Positively Programme

Before starting your day it's important to take a few minutes to really think about what you want from it; that is, to think properly about your desired outcome for the day rather than just going over the same old things, or simply moseying on.

Thinking about the following questions, get into a relaxed and focused state as covered in Chapter Four. Accompany this by taking in some deep breaths through the nose and out through the mouth, energizing your mind and body for the day ahead. Strongly visualize these things and even say them aloud, believe them and take action. For more details on working effectively with goals and outcomes long-term see Chapter Seven.

The Questions:

- What do you want to achieve today?
- What has to happen today for you to have achieved this?
- What can you do today to take steps towards achieving your ultimate goal?

Become that Master Reframer – Seeing Negative Stuff Differently

Look at how you can turn negative situations on their head. This isn't to say that bad or negative things don't happen; rather that, if it does, you can look at what you can do about it by viewing things differently and looking for alternative meanings. You can do this by:

- Looking for the positive in a situation.
- Looking at how you can be proactive.
- Considering all the alternatives to a situation or the next best option.
- Looking at someone's intention for whatever they've done rather than concentrating on their behaviour.
- Finding humour in the situation.
- Taking a philosophical view. What can you constructively learn from the situation?

Reframing situations is something I have had to work on mastering from a young age, and I can attest that it certainly helps keep you keep a strong state of mind, even when negative things happen.

For example, a few years back I remember having such a severe hypo (very low blood sugar level) early one Sunday morning that I went into violent fits; it took several strong people to steady me. I was in bed, in my birthday suit, perspiring and shaking uncontrollably. The fits were so strong that I had to be given a rectal diazepam (a minor tranquillizer). I came round to find my partner and three paramedics standing over me in my bedroom. Hmmm. If there was ever a time I could have felt embarrassed, and feared dying in my sleep, that was it! The violent convulsions went on for some time, too, so I was pretty exhausted (I've had far less tiring workouts in the gym!).

But rather than looking at this episode as embarrassing, and thinking that I should sit around all day recovering or dwell on it – and risk manifesting a fear of sleeping – I quickly reframed the situation by joking about the great show I'd just given the paramedics. We all had some tea and some normal conversation for a bit, partly to reassure the paramedics that I was fine, but it was also a good chance for everyone to recover after such an intense situation. The reality of what the paramedics had just done for me outweighed any potential embarrassment, too, not to mention the fact that I still had my life – this was all the more reason to focus on embracing it.

Afterwards, I reflected and positively focused on the fact that I was alive and well, reframing further as I took all the positive learnings from what was a potentially grave situation.

Ensure You're Surrounded by Positive Influences

It's well known that the people and environment around us have a massive impact on how we think, feel and behave; to the point that it can be the difference between make or break. If we hang around someone or something long enough, we often become like them. It's therefore massively important to make sure we're surrounded by positive, supportive, encouraging and successful people and environments with a healthy mindset and atmosphere, because this breeds and rubs off. Negativity, too, spreads like wildfire, as mentioned earlier. This is something we often see in the workplace and it can lead to a very poor working environment where people survive rather than thrive!

The most positive, successful and healthy types of people tend to mix with the same sort of groups. Bear this in mind in order to support yourself in the best way possible; fear only breeds fear – remember the example in Chapter Four about two agoraphobics living together?

Lose Your Inhibitions – They Serve No Positive Purpose

Inhibitions pertain to a deep-rooted fear of something. We've seen already that fear, unless it is a natural fear or the protective "fight-or-flight" response, serves no purpose; therefore, inhibitions only hold us back. Chapters Four to Eight particularly offer resources to support you to become aware of any personal inhibitions and limitations you may have and let them go. This will enable you to dramatically improve your life and help you achieve your real goals, moving further toward zone zero.

Embrace Your Mistakes

Never fear making mistakes, dwell on them or over-generalize from them; this will only ever limit you. If we never make a mistake, it tends to mean we are never trying anything new. In fact, we need to make mistakes in order to learn. Constructively learning from our mistakes allows us to successfully move on and avoid making the same error more than once.

Have a Great Belief System

One of the most important things we can ever do if we really want something is to wholeheartedly believe in what we want and in everything we do and have the courage of our convictions. This way we'll always achieve our goals, because we'll have the motivation, drive and persistence to stick with things until we get exactly what we want. There are always bumps and challenges in life, but we'll have the tenacity and patience needed to see things through and find solutions that will get us where we want to go. In this respect, patience and persistence, plus a strong belief in ourselves, really do pay off.

Having a great belief system is about what we deep-down expect for ourselves and therefore what we attract. Do you believe you deserve good things? Do you believe you are "really" worthy or good enough? Or do you believe you have to struggle and things need to be complicated to have value? Or that you need to go through challenges before you're allowed success? Or that you have to "graft" to make money?

If any of the above statements resonate deep down, you need to work on having enough self-awareness to dig deep, get to the root and sort this out. Chapters Six to Eight will help with this.

Be Thankful

Make a list of all the things you are grateful for in your life. This will always help to positively shift your mindset and, in line with the physical workings of the universe, you'll begin attracting more of these things.

Be Free to Be You

Avoid labelling: "gay", "transgender", "vegan", "coeliac", "anxious", "diabetic" ... and so on. Just because you may have displayed a behaviour, condition, thinking or emotion for a long time doesn't mean it is static and can't be changed. Remember it all starts with a thought!

There are so many things in life we can fear and, professionally speaking, I see many people who fear being themselves because of having had horrible experiences; but the key is to let these experiences make you rather than break you and refuse to let them hijack or define you. It makes your focus wrong; that experience and that label can consume you and detract from you just being you. If anyone else has a problem with you, it really is their problem because it ultimately pertains to something they either don't like about themselves or couldn't handle themselves – or even indicates that you are someone or have done something they want to, but feel unable to. Or, simply, something about you conflicts with

THEIR values. There is nothing you can do or need do about this; so, enjoy being you and go for it!

Think Outside the Box to Adapt and Overcome

Be resourceful and flexible so that you can find other ways to achieve the same outcome and get exactly what you want. Explore every avenue you can think of. There is always more than one way to do something and nothing ever needs to stop you, especially irrational fear or deep-rooted limitations.

It can help to think outside the box by taking one idea and asking, "What is this an example of?" and then "What is another example of this?" This should soon generate and lead to other ideas.

Value All Your Experiences and Create Wisdom

It's so important to value all our experiences, because they shape who we are, what we know and who we become.

Whether they're good, bad or indifferent at the time, our experiences are how we learn, and our character influences what we do with this. It's important to keep learning; it means we keep evolving and, above all, living. If we don't keep learning and experiencing new things with an open mind, we won't develop, grow and open new opportunities. Instead, we'll get left behind and wilt away.

Some experiences, obviously, aren't good; but we can still express the negative emotion a bad experience creates in as short a period of time as possible and let it go to the extent that we can look back on it without the negative emotional charge. In this way it simply becomes wisdom. If you can find the positive learnings and be aware of the new resources you can take from the experience, this will always enable you to move forward in life.

Be Confident and Aware, Never Complacent

It's important to be confident and keep a positive focus, but at the same time to be aware of everything around us, to protect us from becoming complacent. Complacency only leads to mistakes and serves no positive purpose. Confident awareness is the key – thinking and planning with a positive focus to ensure we achieve our desired results.

Problem-Solve

Seeing yourself as a solution strategist and valuing that ability in yourself is a great way to think about and utilize fear. In my experience in professional practice, helping people overcome fear means helping them to also recognize some of the unique resources they have gained from using their fear. This often involves unique, creative, independent and resourceful ways of thinking. Valuing these abilities in yourself, and making the most of them, can help you create some positives from your old fear and provide you with some great skills for the future. For example, with my old fear of heights I definitely stretched my creative thinking skills to make up some of the avoidance strategies I came up with, negotiating different outcomes and finding new alternatives.

Be Proactive: "Do – Don't Dwell"

Avoid focusing on what's wrong, or what you or anyone else thinks something *should* be; instead, concentrate on what you can do and what you actually want to happen ultimately. Whatever you choose to focus on, you will attract much more of it back to you, so avoid dwelling on any intense bad feelings; don't indulge them – unless you want more!

Have a Mindful Philosophy

Whatever happens in life – amazing, good, bad, tragic or indifferent – there's always something we can positively learn from it, and it can always play a greater purpose in our lives. If we learn to look at what we can positively take from life's challenges, it can enable us to learn the lessons we need in order to develop our resources and successfully move on.

Consider the Emotional Body

It can be easy to dismiss the idea that emotions have an effect on our health, but they do, and dramatically too! Whether we start with feeling irritation, impatience, criticism, jealousy, bitterness, resentment, frustration, anxiety, nervousness, tension, worry, doubt, insecurity . . . they are all emotions that pertain to fear and they all poison the body.

Learning to be aware of negative emotions, letting them go, finding resolution and taking positive learnings from them will allow the body's organs to function properly and avoid creating the negative effects that manifest as ill health (as discussed in Chapter Three). Being more aware of any negative emotions and letting them go will significantly improve health, physically, psychologically and emotionally, in both the short and the long term.

Let Go of Fear for the Right Reasons

Choose to let go of fear in order to be free and live a fulfilled, happy, healthy life rather than because of everything it prevents you from doing and the harm it can cause. Doing this will create a much more positive focus and is in line with concentrating on what you positively want. This is important because what we focus on, we get, so we want to be strongly, and predominantly, positive! It will make achieving your goals much easier.

Conversely, positively enjoy and embrace the fear that does you no harm – the rush effect. It's the fine line between pain and pleasure. For example, if I'm doing something like queuing for a very high, vertical-drop roller coaster or I'm about to go on stage and talk to a room full of hundreds of people, or jump out of a plane – I feel sick with nerves but I allow myself to feel them because I love the adrenaline rush and the euphoric effect I get from it afterwards.

Dare to Be Open-Minded

Always have an inquisitive mind when looking for the answers you want. Be willing to ask yourself whether you've got anything to lose by keeping an open mind, applying fresh ideas and freeing yourself from criticism and doubt. Closing your mind to possibilities only creates limitations and negative emotions, which in turn lead to ill health – the opposite of everything we want!

The minute we take something negative at face value, thus surrendering our independent thought and a host of potential opportunities, we are at the mercy of negative emotions. Imagine how depressed I could have been if I gave in to the common fear – and an actual diagnosis – of going blind from diabetes. Instead I confronted the fear and took action to do something about it, uncovering a whole new world with infinite opportunity. And now I enjoy full eyesight and more to the point metaphysically speaking, everything I see!

Explore the Unconventional or Different

Have the courage to explore, understand and use unconventional ideas to make new and exciting discoveries. Often it is unconventional ideas that provide us with the best solutions, so never be afraid to investigate these.

The more we explore, discover and learn, the more neural networks we build in our brain, which increases our capacity to think and develop. This is yet another of the factors that enables us to grow as people. Moreover, if we keep growing and personally evolving in this way, we progress to a new level of consciousness and, to quote Einstein once more: "No problem can be solved from the same level of consciousness that created it."

Hence, we need to have an open mind to learn new things and think differently – especially when it comes to our fears and how far we can travel to break free from them.

Have a Great Sense of Humour – Laugh Whenever You Can!

Being willing to laugh is important for great health and for making everything we have to confront in life that much easier. It helps us to appreciate that life is for living, in the sense that it generates endorphins and powerful biochemicals in the brain to counteract those induced by fear; and as endorphins are the body's endogenous morphine, it acts as a natural pain-reliever too.

The 25 Markers of a Zone-Zero Personality

The following markers are consistent with the mindset of people who display a zone-zero personality: essentially the personality of a person who seems to get or have everything they want in life. It's therefore useful to see which attributes you already display, which you display less of and those which you think you could positively accentuate more:

- Shows a distinct lack of inhibitions.
- Appears naturally positive, optimistic and open-minded.
- Has an unshakable belief system.
- Displays independent and innovative thought.
- Has naturally high energy levels and enthusiasm.
- Is purposeful and pragmatic, driven by results and a broader positive intent.
- Is happy to lead and experiment, trusting themselves.

- Encourages, empowers and inspires others.
- Is a natural problem-solver: nothing has to be a problem or drama.
- Has a flexible, dynamic and amenable approach to life.
- Often displays different or unconventional ways of doing things.
- Embraces change, new opportunities and creativity.
- Will go with the flow where possible.
- Enjoys calculated risks and thrill-seeking adventure.
- Is self-reliant, dedicated, resourceful and responsible.
- Is persistent, resilient and undeterred.
- Has a firm life philosophy and rises above what others think.
- Has high self-awareness and is very intuitive.
- Is calm in a crisis and gets on with things with little fuss; solution-focused.
- Focuses on what they "can do" and "do want".
- Puts well-being, fulfilment and enjoyment before winning.
- Never fears failure or getting things wrong.
- Can handle uncertainty by trusting in the process of life – has a metaphysical, quantum approach to life (see Chapter Eight).
- Displays great tenacity – if they want something, they will find a way to get it or do it and know that they will.
- Appreciates and loves life irrespective of what their current situation is – trusting that it is part of the process and it is happening for a reason, providing opportunity to push them forward.

Mindset is what really makes a difference. Whatever you really want, it's all out there waiting for you. It's every individual's choice as to how far to take this. Working carefully through the rest of this book will provide everything you need to do so.

> *"Mindset is everything. It determines our character, the paths we choose, and the results we get in life."*

Summary

- By utilizing the contents of this chapter, the resources throughout the book and your own great attributes, you'll always ensure an indestructible mindset fit for maximum success, whatever challenges life may bring.

CHAPTER SIX

BREAKING BOUNDARIES: ULTIMATELY RELEASING FEAR AND ANXIETY

N ot all fears involve spiders or going up gigantic buildings, or even speaking to large crowds of people. They may instead be of a completely different, intangible nature, things like an irrational fear of death or anxiety that leads someone to have compulsive dangerous thoughts, or intense worry about getting ill.

In this case, for releasing purely psychological fears as opposed to practical fears, we just have to work a bit differently. We also need a slightly different evidence procedure – the way we ultimately test to check if you've really conquered your fear; obviously I'd never recommend testing out getting a serious medical diagnosis, dying or carrying out compulsive dangerous acts to provide evidence you're no longer scared of such!

We often also need to have done enough mental preparation and procedures to even get to the point of being ready to release our deepest fears. For example, just being able to talk about something can form a large part of overcoming the fear itself. Applying all the steps in Chapter Four will greatly help in reaching this stage.

In any case, no matter what your specific fear, anxiety or limitation may be and irrespective of whether it has manifested physically or psychologically, there are multiple ways to release it once and for all. You may find some of the points and resources in this chapter work better for you than others; however, there is something here to help everyone, ranging from useful practical knowledge and support to deep fear-release techniques.

You may have always had background anxiety without being sure why and without addressing it; or think you are "just an anxious person". In either scenario you may well have found it safer to stay in your comfort zone; but there could be physical or medical contributors to your anxiety that need addressing. Below are some physical examples of where, why and how other types of anxiety can arise, as well as one particular case highlighting how anxiety can be so strongly suggested to a person that it is created where it didn't and shouldn't exist.

However, if you still have any doubts over your anxiety, please be sure to consult your medical doctor.

A Game of Hide and Seek

Anxiety, especially background anxiety, can often be attached to certain chronic medical conditions but it's not always obvious when you become accustomed to living with something for a long time. Anxiety in this respect, can sometimes exist as a symptom of the condition, as well as, in general because of everything the condition entails.

For example, I know from much personal experience how living with Type 1 diabetes can cause anxiety in general – through things like repeated hospital visits, blood tests, judgement, personal safety, and potential complications, as well as the coexisting anxiety that is an actual symptom of blood sugars running too low. Asthma, epilepsy and many other chronic conditions can produce very similar issues surrounding anxiety too, so it's important to be mindful of these and make the relevant distinctions to best eliminate or reduce it. This is important because such elements can be easily dismissed yet potentially be subconsciously holding you back from breaking out of your comfort zone.

You can of course also investigate and explore specific ways to help with anxiety related to these conditions if they affect you. There are some very helpful techniques and resources set out in my previous book *Mind Body Diabetes*; and note that they are widely applicable and can be of use in other chronic conditions too.

Anxiety Alerts – When Anxiety Is Telling You To Focus

There are also a host of physical factors, termed "medical mimics",[6] that are a medical underlying root of feelings of anxiety and, more broadly, various psychological and emotional symptoms that leave you not quite feeling yourself. It's therefore exceptionally important to listen to your body. If any of the following resonates with you and you are unable to find a link to any particular root triggers for your anxiety through everything otherwise discussed, or it doesn't change, you should consult your doctor as soon as possible to rule out any of these "medical mimics". If you're feeling below par then you must focus on treating this first to allow yourself to then distinguish, for real, any fears and limitations you have that may be preventing you from moving out of your comfort zone.

Nutrition

We will look at nutrition and diet in more depth later on, but it's important to note now that any malnutrition, vitamin deficiency, malabsorption or an excess of vitamins can mimic an array of emotional conditions.

Deficiency in the B vitamins and in iron, for example, can result in symptoms of anxiety and sometimes panic attacks, as has been found in a clinical research study from Japan. The study concluded that those participants who had a shortage of both vitamin B6 and iron experienced periodic anxiety attacks, which were marked by episodes of hyperventilation.[7]

Hormones

Hormones are chemical messengers that tell different parts of the body what to do, and an imbalance in their presence in the body can result in symptoms including anxiety. Conditions such as thyroid disorders can be responsible for anxiety symptoms such as a high heart rate, high blood pressure, palpitations or tremors, in some cases feeling like a panic attack.

As many women will tell you, perimenopause and the menopause itself can lead to extremely intense feelings of anxiety, caused at least in part by levels of the hormones oestrogen and progesterone.

Infectious Conditions

Some infectious conditions such as Lyme disease are sometimes associated with various psychiatric symptoms including anxiety.

Tumours

Many tumours cause a host of psychiatric symptoms. And, although this is rare, certain tumours[8] produce adrenaline, which can cause unexplained anxiety.

Head Trauma

Even mild head trauma can cause unexplained anxiety, and sometimes some time after the trauma was sustained, which makes it harder to relate the anxiety to the incident.

Other Conditions

Wilson's disease (a genetic condition) interferes with the metabolism of copper levels in the body; if left untreated it[9] can cause, among many symptoms, intense feelings of unexplained anxiety; unfortunately I know exactly how intense this can get: I personally have experienced it. It is however, thankfully, a pretty rare condition.

Medication and Other Factors

All medications can have side-effects and these include in some cases anxiety. Homeopathic remedies, stimulants such as too much caffeine, illegal drugs and alcohol withdrawal can also produce these kind of symptoms.

Anxiety and Mistaken Identity

Sometimes what we think of and label as anxiety might in fact be our mind and body alerting us to something that's just not quite right, a signal for us to focus and pay attention to something. This "something" may be either a problem in the physical body as discussed above or an issue we detect unconsciously in our external environment.

The following case, as documented by my client Jasmine, is a very profound example of anxiety being misunderstood for years and the devastating repercussions.

> Had you asked me or my family this time last year whether I thought it'd ever be possible for me to live my life free from anxiety and medication I'd have told you no way, impossible! Simply because, for as long as I can remember, we'd been told it was the only way I would be able to function day to day and live a "normal" life. I was just an anxious person. However, I saw it as being better than constantly feeling anxious and vulnerable to serious bouts of depression over a feeling I couldn't understand.

Ever since I started school I had been labelled "an anxious child", and had been prescribed medication not typically given to children that I was told would keep me on a level where I could live free from anxiety and what was later labelled "depression". At my worst times I was unable to leave my house for months and felt that life wasn't worth living. These feelings would just get more intense, resulting in crippling emotions and inevitably spiralling into depression. I was seriously desperate and my family even more so because they had to keep me going; I was ready to give in.

My medical team introduced various new medications. However, I suffered extreme reactions to the majority of them; yet the seeming answer was my team adding new medication to take away the side-effects! It was just a cycle; but at the time it made sense to me, and anyway why would my family or I question the medics and my mental health team?

I was referred to multiple psychiatrists and counsellors, all of whom told me my anxiety and depression had a root cause, and that I was to think hard about what this could be. I was even told at one point that I was suffering PTSD, although the traumatic event in question remained a mystery to me – I could think of nothing. And the fact I couldn't identify anything just made me feel even worse. What the hell was wrong with me?

Eventually, aged 17 I was admitted to a psychiatric unit, a very small unit where the places were strictly for people suffering the most severe mental health disorders. I couldn't understand it. What was so wrong with me that I needed to be admitted here for a six-week stay? It was as if no one knew what else to do with me.

Being in this environment obviously took its toll on me and my anxiety worsened to the point where I discharged myself. Following that, I was passed on to the adult mental health services, where I was told to continue taking increased medication. I was in knots, feeling constantly in a black hole. I could make no sense of it.

Eventually my mum reached a point of despair and, not knowing what else to do, found the Pinnacle Practice, who were certain they could help. She arranged for me to see Dr Em. Initially I was very reluctant: I was in the middle of a very low period and could not believe this would be any different from the many other professionals I'd seen before. I was in no frame of mind to start again on the same old methods I'd previously been taught.

However, I couldn't have been more wrong and at this point my life was to change beyond recognition. I was confronted with an entirely different way of thinking and a whole new understanding of my experience and feelings that was completely alien to me. However, the things Dr Em said were the only things that had ever resonated, and something changed deep inside me; I had a surge of positive energy and it was an amazing feeling!

It took me some time to even comprehend the prospect of being medication-free because of everything I'd ever been told. Not to mention medication had been my safety net for 11 years, so it was terrifying – but I knew I could do this.

I left my first session feeling a sudden energy. A real positive energy. I'd never before been to any session where I'd been asked what I actually wanted in life. Never had I spoken about positive outcomes – or any outcome at all for that matter.

After a few sessions I realized I really needed to put all of my efforts into breaking out of my comfort zone. I needed to put my trust in what we were working on and invest my energy in realizing my true self.

Thank goodness I did because now, after six months, I am – amazingly – completely free from medication. I am a confident, happy 23-year-old and finally feel I am "my true self". I have learned to believe in myself and trust my own decisions, and that anxiety is not always what it seems and was never really the problem!

It's something I never imagined would happen, and I didn't realize how much I wanted it to happen until I began this journey. I finally know that my life will never be limited again by the feelings that come with the anxiety and depression that were eventually created for me for real from the fear of being sectioned, never knowing up to this point what was wrong with me, and the absolute fear of reacting to more medication. Em has shown me that, even when life seems unbearable and you have been led to believe you'll just always be that way, there's always something that can be done!

Jasmine Doughty

I had read carefully through Jasmine's medical notes and personal history and nothing ever struck me as particularly alarming, yet she had been given the working diagnosis of "Mixed Anxiety and Depressive Disorder". This was a diagnosis considered severe enough to warrant hospitalization and an expected lifetime of unpleasant medication – and yet to me things did not add up. I observed from Jasmine's notes that she'd been tried on most of the different medications on offer and either had a severe reaction or bad side-effects with them all. This straight away signalled to me that her body was most likely rejecting the medication, and as time went on I suspected this was because she currently didn't need medicating for this "anxiety" (and never really had).

In our first session Jasmine asked me what I thought was wrong with her. I replied:

"In actual fact – absolutely nothing!"

I explained to Jasmine that I thought she simply had a more heightened awareness than is usual, which made her more receptive and sensitive to experiences and people.

When this heightened awareness (or hyperalertness, to give it another name) detected something looming, it presented itself as a feeling of anxiety, like radar signalling to her to question what was really going on as I suspected she was deeply intuitive. I suggested to Jasmine that she work on embracing this as a gift and learning how to positively work with it and react to it.

I also helped Jasmine to see that because no one until now had recognized this, she had been almost primed to think she was this "anxious, depressive person". Therefore, she'd naturally fallen into a comfort zone of sorts, learning to expect a certain negative pattern and subsequently reacting accordingly, in a cycle, when in fact this wasn't her "true" life's blueprint at all and she had never been living the life she should have. This explained her apathy – or "depression", as it had been labelled – about the life she was currently living.

I also explained that it was quite natural to be in this "induced" state because she had created feelings of despair in reaction to everything that had been suggested to her, the fear of being sectioned and never understanding herself, not to mention the fear of more medication and possible severe reactions to it.

When I explained all this to Jasmine, it was as if a physical weight was suddenly lifted off her shoulders; the most fantastic and visible change as though a light had been switched on – the surge of energy she describes above!

Our sessions continued and it was a case of putting all of Jasmine's past into perspective, changing her old thought patterns and releasing the attached negative emotional charges she had accumulated from her life experiences. Gradually she learned to reprogramme herself and embrace the "new" Jasmine.

It was also crucial in her success that I help with getting her whole family, social and professional network used to this sudden change and for them to wholeheartedly accept it. In any individual change work like this, it's critical to explain your intentions to the people around you and ensure they are positively on board too, otherwise it can prove to be a very unhelpful negative pull. An individual's support network can be, quite simply, the difference between make or break.

With Jasmine, there was never really an anxiety "disorder" to deal with. However, because she had been labelled as having "anxiety", she had no reason to believe otherwise. So it actually came true.

The brilliant news is that, upon gaining this awareness of her condition, and having an exceptional underlying core mindset to enable her to make these positive changes, Jas was able to break her personal boundaries, step outside of her comfort zone and engage courageously in our process of moving forward. She did so with much dedication and excited energy.

This was big stuff to comprehend and overcome, considering all the traumatic suffering and negative programming she'd been living through for the majority of her life. Yet by thinking differently and establishing an entirely new consciousness, breaking from her old patterns and bucking the trends of what was previously expected and anticipated of her old self, she established her true self, the vibrant, successful young woman she is today.

And, whatever the root of your personal anxiety or limitations may be, you can choose not to accept medical labels; not to mention media sensation, social media trends or celebrity endorsements of conditions. If you do, you are likely to remain in a comfort zone, unable to lead a life beyond limits. If you choose not to, you can, if you so wish, achieve what Jasmine achieved.

Anxiety-Busting

As we now know, anxiety to a greater or lesser extent is just another form of fear, so if we can learn to control anxiety, we can overcome our fears. We can use our brains' neurology to naturally support our ability to self-calm and successfully tackle stress and anxiety to positively move forward and get the best results in whatever we do.

The following discussions and techniques are potentially invaluable in helping you achieve this.

A Metaphysical Approach to Anxiety

The term metaphysics here refers to the root thought patterns and emotional root cause that alter the biochemistry of the brain and lead to physical changes in the body, ultimately manifesting as ill health and numerous physical and psychological conditions. In other words, and as demonstrated on many occasions by scientific studies (I talk about this in *Mind Body Diabetes*) our physical health is only ever a reflection of what we hold in our minds. In terms of anxiety, this ultimately pertains to us not trusting the flow and the process of life. It is simply our mind alerting us that we need to focus in the right direction and pay attention where needed. So the questions are:

- What might we need to do practically to resolve the root of anxiety?
- What might we need to positively learn?

Practically speaking, meditation can help with this process as it can allow you to find the space to resolve your anxiety by relaxing your mind, allowing for the answers to naturally present themselves. We will cover meditation in some detail later on. Certain music that helps slow down your brainwaves to accompany this can also be of great value, as we saw in Chapter Four.

It is also helpful from a metaphysical point of view to counter the root of anxiety by repeating the following mantra whenever you start to feel anxious, at random points throughout the day or during your meditation:

"I trust in the process of life, and I am safe. Relax, release, let go."

In any case, everything has a metaphysical origin (a deep, first root) but it is worth acknowledging that not all roots are necessarily something traumatic. The relevant answers you need to discover are there, buried deep in your mind, and they will present themselves to you consciously when you are ready to let them go fully.

Changing Perspectives

If you, for example, own a business and have some critical and defining decisions to make, such as whether or not to do business with a client you dislike or find difficult, seeing things objectively rather than emotionally will make a great deal of difference to the outcome. Essentially it avoids emotional reasoning.

This simple technique is nonetheless powerful. It instigates a different way of thinking and so can remove the emotional charge that can come with being too personally involved in the event and the moment, unable to see the wood for the trees. It helps you gain perspective and put things into context. It can even help you to find situations quite amusing or trivial; this is because you will have created the distance needed to remove a negative emotional charge, and negative emotions only cloud judgement and perspective. This is similar to when something seemed like a nightmare at the time but later on with hindsight (in this case, time creating the distance needed), you can view it as all quite amusing.

- Sitting or lying comfortably, breathe in through your nose and out through your mouth.
- Relax your arms, shoulders and neck, allowing this feeling of relaxation to spread like a wave throughout your entire body.
- As you experience or think about the stressful event, imagine stepping out of your body and seeing yourself in the scene, as if you were watching it as a movie.
- Then begin to see it as if through another person's eyes. Imagine yourself to be a bystander or watching on CCTV.
- Look at the situation through the eyes of this other person. *Really* step into their shoes.
- Now imagine you are another person again: a neutral individual; perhaps a psychologist, a business consultant, coach or another kind of advisor or analyst of the situation. What advice would you give to yourself?

Note: When changing perspectives, it's important to get fully into the mind and body of someone else. Use all your senses to do this. Delve into their life and their line of thinking (their values too, if you know them). Adopt their posture and mannerisms. Really imagine having their situation.

A good example of when to apply this technique is if a family member is causing you a particular challenge. See them for the *person* they are, rather than the *relationship* you have with them and all the expectations that go with this.

Take a parent, for example. All of us naturally have certain expectations and needs we want met by our parents, so those times when their behaviour fails to match our personal expectations can naturally heighten our emotions, the situation or our anxiety levels. This can then prove distracting or self-limiting.

By *disassociating* (disconnecting) from the family relationship for a moment, and seeing our family members instead as ordinary people, things can start to look and feel very different to us – more rationalized and offering a different perspective on the incident or situation. We can ask ourselves: if they weren't our parents, would things seem as unusual or upsetting? Might their thinking or behaviour even become acceptable? This technique can help us to see things objectively by *desensitizing* us to a personal situation.

Your Root Solution-Set

Whenever you are feeling anxious, ask yourself the following:

- For what purpose am I feeling anxious?

You'll no doubt get a string of reasons, but for every one of those reasons ask yourself further:

- For what purpose? . . . And for what purpose . . .

Keep going with this question to your responses until you get to the real root answers you need.
    Then stop and think for a minute:

- Is the superficial or momentary reason for me being anxious or stressed really going to prevent me from ultimately gaining happiness and fulfilment or achieving my important goals in life? Or is it just an inconvenience that needs a bit of creative thinking, patience and flexibility to overcome it?

Ask yourself how you can be a problem-solver with the issue instead:

- What would you advise someone else faced with such a challenge? Do you have a contingency plan, if needed? What else can you do if "the unexpected thing" should happen?

Whatever the answer may be, it's important to make the decision to take personal responsibility for your own life and look to:

- What you can do about it and how best you can manage something, rather than worrying about or wasting time on what you can't do or what won't happen.

Importantly, there's a big difference between "focus" and "awareness", and it's crucial to be mindful that we need both.
    Our focus is where our energy and attention are predominantly directed; however, our awareness is what keeps us mindful of all else going on in our life, enabling us to remain responsible and safe as we focus on the right things.

This way we can see beyond the fear, stress and anxiety and keep our mind on what counts; so all that we do want will come to us a lot easier and quicker.

- In a nutshell, focus on what you do want, rather than on what's wrong.

Get used to finding the positives of a situation and how you can move forward from it. Although at times this can be challenging things you can constructively learn. Just have a good search and think outside the box.

Always ask yourself:

- What message is life trying to give you, how can you overcome obstacles and what it is you are really working towards?
- What is your real intention, beyond the immediate stress/anxiety/fear?

Keep your focus on this answer because, as we have discussed already, what you wholeheartedly focus on, you will attract back. So if you home in on the negative things, you'll attract more negativity back to you, and the cycle will only continue – this gives rise, incidentally, to the common belief that things happen in threes or "It's just one thing after the other."

From experience, I'm sure you already know that if you deep-down expect something, it happens . . . We programme ourselves to fulfil this by either consciously or unconsciously giving that expectation our attention and devotion. We then get it back – good, bad or indifferent. If you expect to get stressed about something you likely will, because you're focusing on the wrong things. Work to change this and instead to focus positively on your intention for doing something by using the above questions and considering other ways to reach your positive intention where necessary.

It's important to appreciate, though, that you can't just think something and have it happen! To guarantee you work your own positive law of attraction, see Chapters Seven and Eight, because once you fully grasp this principle and work it in your favour, it really is one of the most powerful tools you can ever possess, in every aspect of your life!

Awareness and Reprogramming

It's important to be able to recognize when you might be starting to feel stressed and anxious, so that you can apply the above techniques. Notice what happens in this situation:

- Is there a specific feeling?
- Do you experience a physical reaction, such as stomach ache, headache, extreme tiredness, toilet trouble?
- Does your behaviour change?
- Do you shout or cry easily?

If you struggle to recognize changes, it may help to:

- Keep a trend diary – a regular diary of your feelings. Look for any patterns and triggers that you need to work on to eliminate or address the root problem; you may be unaware of this consciously and only realize it when it's written in black and white.
- Similarly, if you are close to someone and trust them, you could ask them to gently point out any little changes in your behaviour they notice when you begin to get stressed.

Keep a Sense of Humour

The more we can avoid taking ourselves too seriously the better! The more things we can find to laugh at and the better we can become at whatever makes us laugh and feel good, whether it's "poking fun", "friendly banter" or anything else, the more we will be able to relax.

Humour and laughing alter our physical state. The release of endorphins (feel-good brain chemicals) triggers more positive thoughts and feelings. This in turn allows us to focus more easily on what we *can do* to resolve our stresses, rather than focusing on the problem, which only results in bad feelings, hinders our thought process and contributes to more stress.

Things that can help:

- Someone else really exaggerating you displaying fear. This won't work for everything fear-related but, in some situations, it can help very much. It helps you to see your behaviour and how you might want to change it.

For example, I mentioned in the preface that I once got stuck on a rope bridge, crying and frozen. Whenever I attempt something similar now, my partner does an impression of this scene. It always makes me laugh and changes my state.

- Laughing and making a conscious effort to smile to change your mood.

Try thinking of something sad or infuriating while smiling! Keep in mind the expression on your face and your body language – these are inextricably linked, as discussed in Chapter Two. It is hard to smile or laugh when you aren't thinking of something positive, so make a conscious effort to watch your facial expressions, tone of voice and body language – mind and body profoundly affect one another. Find something to help; personally I like to watch something I find really funny, like clips from sitcoms.

- Pretending to smile or be calm and happy. This will even help alter your mood and lead to clearer thinking, which will help you solve the problem causing you stress in the first place. Pretending to be, or doing an exaggerated impression of, someone who is either overly comical or very calm can also really help to get you into that state.

British comedian Lee Mack performs a great sketch about him and his wife singing an argument in a musical-theatre style so the kids wouldn't realize they were arguing. Apart from being hilarious, it shows how changing your thinking and feelings about something can lessen the negative impact, stress and anxiety and make things seem comical, different and less serious. At the very least it can help you to relax a little by articulating things in a different way or just expressing some negative energy. By doing this, your state of mind begins to alter. Have a go. It does work!

Emotional Restart

Fully immersing your head in either warm or cold water for a few seconds is said to reset the amygdala (the part of the brain that deals with emotion). This can change your focus to a more positive one; with a clearer head, you can begin to see things differently. This will help give you the serenity and fresh, clear thinking needed to confront the root cause of the stress in a new way, so you can do something proactive about it. It's also useful if you want to alter your state after a challenging day and before you go to sleep.

Take a Two-Minute Timeout

Another simple technique, but never underestimate it. It is very effective and (obviously!) doesn't take a lot of time.

- Start by sitting down to do some deep breathing. Use the "ocean breath" technique from Chapter Four: inhale deeply through your nose and exhale deeply through your mouth. Imagine you are fogging a mirror with your mouth very slightly open. Do this five times.

- Now, close your eyes and remember your favourite place—a place where you were relaxed, calm and having a good time. Perhaps this was a lovely holiday or a day off work or school. Just indulge for a few minutes. See what you saw, hear what you heard and really feel again those calm, relaxed, fun feelings.

- Alternatively, if you created a positive resource anchor earlier, apply that now; or use your gratitude rock.

Have a go at the "unwinding motion" technique. This will help to bring back some calmness and help you think more clearly by changing your state of mind. This technique activates the mind–body connection by using all your senses to create positive changes.

- Take the time to stop for a minute. Close your eyes and ask yourself where in your body you are carrying the stress, nerves or anxiety you are feeling. Give it a colour, a size and a shape.

- Now shrink the area down, seeing it get smaller and smaller until so small it's able to travel through your body to an exit point, such as your hand (so you can open it up and throw it), your foot to kick it, or maybe your mouth or nose to exhale or blow it out.

- As it's travelling to the exit point, see the colour getting increasingly faint, and as it becomes fainter and fainter, feel the stress, nerves or anxiety becoming less and less intense.

- Now take this small, faded shape and release it from your body, so that you fully release it and let it go. See it drift into oblivion. Physically feel the release.

- Now, have a good stretch and shake it out. As the feeling of stress and anxiety releases, retune your focus, and do everything necessary to tackle the real root cause of this particular anxiety to ensure it stays away for good!

Questions for Yourself

Regularly revisit this list of questions, set out in Chapter Four. They really help to gain positive perspective.

Engage in Regular Activity and Take Yourself out of the Situation

When you are feeling anxious, activity may be the last thing on your mind. At such times, though, it can help enormously if we push ourselves to engage with regular daily activities to normalize situations, providing a different focus and perspective along with more social interaction for distraction. Also, engaging in physical exercise is greatly beneficial; not only does it often address the factors just mentioned, it also helps release those crucial endorphins, the brain's happy chemicals, as well as its natural painkiller endogenous morphine. Physical activity also helps to dilute and work off any built-up stress – remember that excess cortisol and adrenaline? – putting it to better use.

- Make sure the activity is something you enjoy, and which will encourage and motivate you. It could be just a short walk to a coffee shop, sexual activity; walking to your newsagents or post office instead of driving, or parking a distance away from the supermarket entrance to walk a bit further . . .
- Never underestimate the power of fresh air, changing your environment and surrounding yourself with positive people to free your mind and generate endorphins.
- Even just picking up the newspaper, reading a magazine or a good book or calling a friend can be a great distraction to help readjust your focus and take yourself away from the immediate situation.
- Often being in the same environment that the stress or anxiety is created in, or in which it is experienced, causes an automatic association between the two – like the anchors or triggers we have discussed. Therefore, it will always be more challenging to solve a problem and feel differently if you feel confined to, or stuck in, the same environment as the stress or source of anxiety. So it's vital to break out and free ourselves metaphorically as much as physically whenever we can!

Explore and Engage in Meditation

One great way to take yourself out of a situation is to meditate regularly. There are many ways to meditate, so just explore and find your preferred method. It's important that you avoid getting caught up in the specifics of different meditation methods and obsessing over details. All forms of meditation help reduce stress and anxiety, and benefit overall health. Scientific studies have shown that regular meditation can:

- Lower blood pressure and improve circulation.
- Increase energy and creativity.
- Strengthen the immune system.
- Release stress, anxiety, fatigue and toxins.
- Lower blood glucose levels.
- Extend our life by approximately ten years.
- Aid in looking and feeling more youthful.
- Provide more psychological rest than a full night's sleep in just 30 minutes' meditation.
- Aid decision-making and productivity.

So again, don't worry about which meditation method you choose; if it feels beneficial and helpful, then it's right for you. Just be sure to keep your spine as straight as possible to allow for the free flow and unblocking of energy. You can do this by lying on your back on a yoga mat, for example, or sitting in a firm chair with back support, against a wall or supported by cushions to ensure you are comfortable, whether sitting or lying.

There are many meditations to be found on Brainsync.com.

Tackle the Root Cause of Your Anxiety

While the previous techniques we've discussed are invaluable, it is vital to work on getting to the root cause of your anxiety, limitations or fear and fully understand what it's all about so you can let it go for good, because ultimately that will phenomenally transform your life. The following techniques will now deeply assist with this.

If you're struggling to get to the bottom of things and to find your root cause, invest in seeing a good therapist who can assist you in this and help you release the problem or negative emotion once and for all. Although this can feel like a daunting prospect, it's well worth it if you work with the right practitioner for you.

Confront the Problem

Even when other people are involved, it is still our responsibility as the person experiencing the anxiety to look at what it is *we* can do to control and positively change the situation.

The person with the most flexible behaviour in doing this always controls the situation, because they are willing to adapt and use whatever appropriate resources necessary to get the best results.

For example, if your anxiety is to do with undue pressure from your boss at work, confront him or her and make your feelings clear, but always state your ultimate intentions for doing so.

For instance, if the boss is making unnecessary demands by micromanaging you to do extra work and bring in more money for the company, resulting in you feeling so stressed and anxious you require time off, this would defeat the intention; sick days are expensive and cost money rather than make more money.

In such a situation, you might say: "I'm feeling very stressed about your current demands, which is leading to me feeling unwell. Unfortunately, this will result in me needing time off work if it continues. This obviously won't help anyone and runs counter to your initial intention, which was the source of my stress and anxiety in the first place. I am fully aware of your intention, so if I can just get on with my work as productively as possible, it will serve us all best and any additional help in the interim would be greatly appreciated."

If you still feel you're not being listened to, look to what else *you* can do. Have you considered changing companies, working for yourself, a change of career, studying something new, getting what you need to enter management yourself? Either way, use all your resources to confront the problem to solve it.

Separating a person's intention from their behaviour is always useful in any context, whether this is to help the process of appeasement when needing to confront a problem or to better understand a person's behaviour to find a more desirable solution.

For instance, when one of my clients was 15 she was repeatedly arrested for shoplifting (obviously an undesirable behaviour) and simply deemed to be "rogue". However, her ultimate intention for repeatedly doing this was that she was looking after four younger siblings alone and didn't have enough money to feed them otherwise (a very positive intention). So although she could easily be judged "rogue" by the Police, other authorities, general society or future employers, focussing on her intention rather than her behaviour can provide a totally different outlook. Rather a more "determined, courageous and caring survivor" than "rogue".

Write It Down or Talk It Through

Writing things down or talking things through with someone helps to externalize things. It can take some weight off your mind, as well as help you see things in a different light. When you see things written down or hear them said back to you, you can even find the answers to your own problem – things often don't seem half as bad as when we just have them whizzing around inside our heads, which can easily distort the reality of a situation, as well as exacerbate feelings of loneliness. Writing things down can prove very cathartic and talking them through both provides validation and can make things seem far less daunting.

Changing the Showreel: Delete Fears and Phobias

When we experience a trauma or any form of distressing situation, it can imprint in our minds and subsequently manifest physically or psychologically as panic attacks, manifested fears that limit us from doing certain things, bouts of illness or post-traumatic stress disorder, potentially destroying our health as well as critically impeding our quality of life.

I have come across several individuals with diabetes who have been in quite a dilemma because they have a needle phobia – a serious problem given the nature of the condition! So, you can see how certain phobias can fairly easily cause a life-threatening challenge or limitation. It's also the case that most phobias relate back in some way to an initial trauma at some point in a person's life.

We can apply certain techniques to help desensitize and decode a trauma or distress – basically, eliminate the old feelings that are related to such experiences so that our minds begin to process them differently. This works by removing the negative charge associated with the negative situation and replacing it with different, positive feelings. We then begin to see our traumatic experiences differently; we attach different associations and meanings to them that prevent the physical and psychological distress of the current phobia from continuing.

To release a phobia or fear, you first need to ask yourself when your phobia first developed and what event it is related to. You may know the answer to this instantly, in which case apply the steps set out in the exercise below. This event is referred to as the root cause/instigating traumatic trigger.

If you are unsure of what the root cause is, this indicates that it is in your unconscious mind. In this case, you can ask yourself very quickly and without thinking about it "What is the root cause that triggered this phobia?" Take the first answer that comes to mind to be true; but I'll note again that you must do this fast, so that you don't start trying to think consciously of an answer.

If you need more support with this or with getting to the real root, you can visit www.dr-em.co.uk for a free audio download version of this technique, consult a hypnotherapist, NLP professional or psychotherapist.

If your particular phobia makes the following release model challenging or uncomfortable, you can instead explore different ways to work on it. You may want to work with releasing fear as your negative emotion in general, using the RACE™ technique we will come to later in this book; otherwise, contact a relevant professional as mentioned.

Answering with the first thing that come to mind if you don't already know consciously:

- Recall the first event that instigated your fear or phobia – your root cause.
  - What was this?
  - Where was this?
  - When was this?
  - What specifically happened?
- Now imagine you are in a cinema. Go into the projector booth at the back of the cinema and see your root cause/trigger event on the big screen; you are merely watching it from the projection booth, behind the glass – with all the editing controls at your disposal; note that now, because you're going to be making good use of them!
- Now make sure the movie is in black and white and run it forward to the most traumatic point.
- Freeze-frame this scene and then white it out. See the picture getting lighter and lighter, brighter and brighter, eventually becoming so bright that you can no longer see anything other than a complete whiteout blank like snow blindness.
- Now run the rest of the movie backward, this time in colour. As you do so, add in some random, bizarre things like:
  - The odd cartoon character.
  - Funny soundtrack (Benny Hill style).
  - Silly TV ad.
  - Your favourite comedian's face or commentary.
  - Strange scents and tastes like fish and chip flavour cookies or baked bean ice cream, candy floss cat food . . .

The idea is to make this as wacky and bizarre as you can!

- Now run the movie forward in black and white, then backward in colour, with your added extras as above, until you no longer feel any old associated negative emotions about it. As you keep going faster and faster, you may find that the images will fade and become harder to access; keep going.
- If you wish to take this further and delete the memory, keep going until you're unable to access the images any more. White the whole thing out as if the projector has broken and the film reel is being destroyed, then decide: "It's no good!" and quickly switch the screen off.

Now remember the last time you couldn't stop laughing or found something so funny you couldn't contain yourself – see what you saw, hear what you heard and feel the feelings you felt. Make it very vivid with lots of positive, funny emotions. Now replace the useless destroyed showreel with your new funny showreel and play it on the big screen.

- Once you have lost the feelings you once had and are feeling positively different – or you may just be feeling numb; this is normal and fine – switch off the projector and come out of the cinema.
- Check how you feel by trying to think about the old event. Do you feel different about it? What do you need to do to assure yourself that it's gone?

If you still feel any negative emotion, keep repeating this process. Or you may decide you need to dig a little deeper and engage in the RACE™ technique later in this book.

Remember, as mentioned above, that you can always think about getting some external professional help.

Reverse Association

This is a highly effective technique but very simple. All you need is a good imagination!

Basically, whatever you might be afraid of, imagine how it feels on the other side. So, let's say you are afraid of a big spider that you need to remove from the bath and help out of the window . . .

Imagine being as small as a spider in a giant house, with a giant hand coming towards you, not knowing what this hand is going to do to you. Not to mention that enormous furry animal that keeps watching you. All you wanted was a safe place to rest and find some food to survive, like anyone else . . .

Now who should be scared?

Similarly, imagine how another person might feel "on the other side". So, if you are afraid of leaving the house or standing up and talking to a group, consider how someone with a physical impediment might feel, or someone with a health condition that can often throw up curveballs: things like needing quick access to the bathroom, a hearing loop, a quiet space, certain foods and so on. The point is, whatever you may feel vulnerable or exposed about, the next person will also have some insecurity they are battling or have been through too.

Outer Space Technique

This technique can really help with putting everything into perspective.

- Relax: breathe deeply and close your eyes.
- Imagine letting go of all earthly concerns and drifting slowly out of your body. Feel yourself nicely drifting through the air, so high you come out of the atmosphere and drift peacefully into space, where you float weightlessly, easily and effortlessly.
- As you look down, you can see Planet Earth. Just observe how minuscule everything is; so tiny that the hugest thing back on Earth seems so insignificant in the grand scale of the observable universe.
- Now imagine you have drifted further out, to the edge of our galaxy, and observe the infinity of outer space. In front of you are so many other planets and stars (there being more stars than there are grains of sand on Earth!). The Earth itself, when you look back, looks like a tiny pinhead.
- Then as you float around and look out at what lies behind you, you can see more and more galaxies. They all form a phenomenal and never-ending multiverse, making Earth and all its goings-on seem so piffling and unimportant in comparison.
- Ask yourself: in the grand scheme of the multiverse, does your fear really pose a problem? Or is it something you can just deal with?
- Let go, release and lose that old concern; right now, up there in space!

- And when you have, just enjoy drifting slowly back down to Earth, relaxed and refreshed as you re-enter your physical body and open your eyes, ready to easily do what you can so easily do – because in the grand scheme of the multiverse, it's actually no big deal! Let the universe work for you. Chapter Eight will explore this further and more specifically.

Creating a Greater Problem

This concept, touched on earlier in the book (in Chapter Four, "Changing How You Think"), is another way of eliminating a problem by contextualizing things to get some perspective. Thinking about and associating into "what could be worse" in your situation can help to minimize or "cancel out" what you once thought was a huge problem.

- Ask yourself "What could be worse, what is really bad?"
- Really imagine this: see what you might see, hear the noises you might hear and feel the emotions of what that would be like. Also observe any tastes and odours present.
- Now think about your original challenge and ask yourself: Really, how is it a problem? Is it anything to which I can't apply my resourcefulness and available resources and sort it?

The Amygdala Freeze™

This technique is about lessening acute negative emotions in order to allow you to fully confront a situation in the first place – such as approaching a therapist before even getting help for your actual problem, or turning up to a work or school meeting before you have to address something really out of your comfort zone. It can help you to do the very thing that scares you or further address a traumatic root cause. A little bit like putting on a bee suit before you go to harvest the honey.

As we know, the amygdala, hidden deep in the middle of the brain, influences our emotional responses. We also know, from research we looked at earlier using PET scan technology, that when we visualize something with enough specific detail and clarity, the unconscious mind cannot tell the difference between what is real and what is not real. Incredibly, this has been shown to be the case in research where some subjects were asked to vividly visualize exercise and others underwent physical exercise; the two groups were[10] found to have burned a similar number of calories.

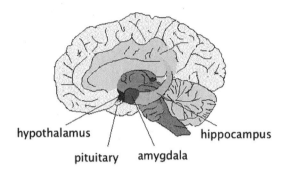

hypothalamus   hippocampus

pituitary   amygdala

It is therefore clear that it's perfectly possible to desensitize or lessen our emotional responses to something through simply visualizing changes to the emotional part of the brain.

- Imagine, with as much detail and clarity as you can, your amygdala deep in the centre of your brain.
- Use whatever image comes to mind (it doesn't matter if this is realistic, as in the image above, or symbolic – just make the imagery vivid and take what comes to you.)
- Observe the size, shape and colour of your amygdala – get specific!
- Now visualize it gradually shrinking until it is about half its current size.
- Change the colour to an icy blue and see your amygdala gradually freeze and harden. For additional "protective" effect, you could even visualize something like tiny miniature men building a solid stone or concrete fortress around your amygdala.
- Now you have created a hardened amygdala, unable to detect additional and superfluous negative emotion that you wish or need to avoid feeling. Remember, all your warm positive emotion is safely protected inside the fortress, along you're your ability to perceive genuine danger. And your positive emotion is so powerfully strong that it will later easily melt the ice and return your amygdala to its original size and shape.
- Now test this by thinking about something that you would ordinarily feel sensitive toward or fearful about and observe your response. Is it less strong than usual? Maybe absent altogether?
- If you feel that your response needs to lessen further, repeat the process, reducing the size of your amygdala and freezing it even further by intensifying the freeze, seeing it getting more and more

solidly frozen as the temperature drops way below sub-zero, until you feel comfortable.

- It's important to remember that your unconscious mind will always protect you and will naturally only restrict unnecessary, negative emotion; you will still feel some emotion, as we all want and need to!
- Once you have become accustomed to successfully dealing with your fear through utilizing this technique, your frozen amygdala will naturally melt and resume back to its original size and shape. Alternatively, you can visualize the reverse of this process happening too.
- To visualize reversing this process, repeat steps 1–3 above. Now visualize your amygdala being subject to a mini brain-heatwave that is causing the ice to melt and your amygdala to get warmer. Give this heat a colour and see it intensify. See your amygdala expanding as it returns to its natural size, shape and colour.

It's also important to note that some of us are naturally more receptive and sensitive to emotion than others; hence the efficacy of this technique is very subjective. Sometimes there may be too much of a deeper underlying emotional root attached that needs resolving and releasing.

In this case you can consult the emotional release work in the RACE™ process below, also accompanied by an audio that you can access at www.dr-em.co.uk.

RACE technique™ – Root Analysis, Cause and Extraction

Get to the "real" root to fully extract and release any fears or limitations.

What's Your Story?

Think about times when you haven't done something that you should have done or don't want to do. Have you ever carefully listened to your own internal dialogue at these times?

Whenever we put things off, avoid doing them or don't have what we want in any context, there's always a deeper reason behind this than we might think – a reason (or a few) behind the reason.

We concoct and tell ourselves stories, creating personal excuses for all kinds of deeper reasons, as you'll come to discover. These stories are so convincing that eventually we come to believe them to be true.

The challenge with this is that we become what we believe . . .

"I haven't got a new job yet because there just don't seem to be any about."

"I just haven't got the time."

"I just don't have the money."

Although there will inevitably be some elements of truth in your story, if you begin to look deeper beneath the surface there will be a reason why this is so; you'll always find underlying reasons, a little like peeling back the layers of an onion.

So what is this really all about? What are the real blockages of energy that are preventing you from attracting more time in your life, or the opportunity of your dream job, or the money to do the things you want to? Because the moment you release these deep unconscious limitations, you WILL begin to attract these things into your life; you'll find that the opportunities to do so suddenly begin to present themselves in line with your true, deep, unconscious belief system.

So to unearth these real reasons that are often lurking buried deep inside – reasons that we are often unaware of consciously – we must ask ourselves what is really behind these reasons we give ourselves for not having all we want right now; and most importantly, why that is so. There will be, at the root, a limiting belief that you have manifested from something that occurred in your past, something that made you at that point unconsciously decide some negative belief. And that something has manifested itself as your limitation.

For instance, when telling ourselves these stories as reasons for not doing something or not having the things we want in life, if we take the example reasons from above, is it more the case that you have the following subconscious beliefs behind them?

"I'm not good enough to achieve . . ."

"I don't really deserve . . . "

"Someone like me can't have that. . . "

"I'll always be like this . . . I'll amount to nothing."

And so on.

Ask yourself: "Is this REALLY the top and bottom of it, or is this about something else?" Push yourself to explore what's really blocking you from doing whatever you might do, or being whoever you could be, and why.

The deeper you go with this, the better the results! Keep probing. Ask yourself why – what do such beliefs really trace back to, what happened in your past for you to form this deep limiting belief? Who or what first put it there? What negative emotions are present when you go back to the root cause event?

Once you can pin down these limitations and fully trace them back to the root cause event and its attached negative emotion, you'll soon discover that the limiting decision you made back in the past is of no substance; in fact it's not even true! From this point you can and you will undo the block that is holding you back and producing the kind of results you currently experience.

If you would like more information and support on doing this, try the free audio "Realizing and releasing limitations" at www.dr-em.co.uk.

Let me share my own personal experience of this.

Since publication of my book about diabetes and how to reverse it, I have avoided getting involved in certain online diabetes communities on which I could promote it.

I know that must sound pretty stupid to anyone else on the face of things. My surface story goes something like this:

"I'm so busy I just never seem to have the time to dedicate to promoting my cause in this way."

Although this is true to a degree, if I really wanted to, I could do it, whether it be late at night or very early in the morning.

So, if I dig a little deeper and ask "So what's REALLY stopping me?", I arrive at something quite different, which then opens up a whole new world, unblocking the energy and pushing me forward in a different way.

In a nutshell, it comes down to a fear of becoming overly immersed in diabetes, maybe to the point where it would be my only focus.

However, going deeper again, I found that the real fear was of being immersed in the negativity and sucked into the black hole of "diabetes doom and gloom".

Essentially, since I was a child I have always been very positive about diabetes and never saw it as a problem; I dealt with any challenges in the best way I could and got on with things. However, since the explosion in social media and the Internet, I have discovered so many incredibly negative ways of thinking about it that I would have never contemplated otherwise – I had therefore been avoiding joining online diabetes communities as I didn't want it to impede my own healing process on a sub- or unconscious level.

However, the paradox of course is that my intention in writing the book was to positively change these negative perceptions with different thinking for different results; to provide something new and exciting.

So, what was the answer?

After revealing the real root problem, through focusing on my highest purpose and intention to begin with – and what I could positively do in the best way possible to achieve this – for me, creating a different medium of communication. Something to establish a more positive, pro-active and real environment. This then gave me the idea of creating a very exciting and practical diabetes well-being expo, something to showcase new innovations and direct attention toward positive change . . . A very productive solution born!

Although that's a very personal example, I hope it highlights how for all of us the surface stories behind our real fears only create even more limitations or blockages about what we really want to achieve and what's truly important.

It comes down to developing a strong awareness of what's behind your internal dialogue and the perpetual reasons you give yourself. You can then begin to explore your deeper roots – peeling the onion to reveal the core so to speak – so you begin to see the paradox in your fear, thus unblocking that energy and revealing the solution by which you will overcome it.

Once you've revealed the real problem you will be able to see which positive resources you need to collect in order to move on and fully release your fear. Once you've done this, you'll find yourself able to take whatever action you need to; you'll do it and never look back – except with a smile about what you have overcome, of course!

To follow is now the critical part of extracting this root that you have established.

The Emotional Extraction Work

It's important to note that your root may not necessarily seem to be from this lifetime as you recall it. Your unconscious mind sometimes works metaphorically so, in this respect, you need to trust what it presents to you and go with it. However or whenever the specific lifetime or period of time is presented to you, it will have major significance as it will ultimately have a relevant attachment to a core negative emotion responsible for the limitations and subsequent blockages of positive energy in your life.

You can use the connected event from your root cause to take valuable positive learnings and resources from it. This is done by observing it from a distance, as if looking through a window, rather than being drawn back into and reliving the negative emotion.

There is help available on this technique in the free audio "Releasing negative emotions" at www.dr-em.co.uk. But it can help to familiarize yourself with the process first; here it is.

- Ask yourself:
  - What was the very first event connected to your specific negative emotion?
  - When was this? How old were you?
  - Was it when you were in gestation? A past life perhaps?
  - Or is it represented in any other context that your mind is presenting to you?
- When you have a clear representation of this time in your mind, observe the connected event, but always from a distance as if you were a bystander watching through a window.
- Begin taking positive learnings from this event (there are always some even when they may seem challenging to find). Notice:
  - What resources have you acquired from this experience?
  - Have you developed any skills from the experience?
  - What else did you positively learn that you otherwise may not have been aware of?
  - What can you utilize and take from this experience to help you going forward in life?
  - How could this experience help you to help or give advice to others?
  - How might this experience have positively influenced your life?
  - Have you met anyone because of your experience that you possibly wouldn't have otherwise and how has this positively shaped your life?
  - What do you need to learn from this event that will allow you to finally release that old attached negative emotion?

Remember, every experience you have without the attached negative emotion becomes wisdom, allowing you to unblock unhealthy energy and make powerful and positive progress. At this point, you will make an enormous psychological leap forward. This is the ultimate positive purpose that you can take from your experience; knowing that it has led you to meet with your ultimate blueprint, allowing you to push forward in life. The new you will therefore be grateful for the experience; for how it has propelled you forward, leading you to now and beyond . . . exciting times!

- Once you feel you have taken all the positive learnings and resources you can from this, take in three very deep, long breaths and expel all that previously attached fear and negative emotion. It has become wholly superfluous to your life.

- Take another objective look at the event and observe how it has changed to being "just an event" with no negative emotional charge ... just wisdom!

If, however, you do still observe any attached negative emotion, then you need to repeat the process to take more positive learnings. Once you have them all, the negative charges will naturally dissipate as they do, visualize obliterating them and seeing them disperse into the atmosphere. This can mean that during the process you may feel numb, emotionally or physically, because you have just released a lot of negative emotion – this is a good thing; your work is still integrating at the unconscious level.

- Observe how you feel. Are there any other events in your life that are associated with this negative emotion? If so, go to these events in your mind one by one and repeat the process, taking all the positive learnings and letting the negative emotion go.
- Once you have finished, come back to now in your mind, and open your eyes. Stretch it out and take some more long deep breaths. Remember to drink plenty of water as you go about your business to flush out the old manifested toxins as you let everything integrate and relax back into the new you – a fun, exciting and fearless personality ready to go forth and achieve all you can!

Remember, you can download free audio versions of all the main techniques mentioned in this chapter at www.dr-em.co.uk.

Eat Away Your Fear

You might be surprised to learn that what you eat can make an enormous difference in terms of increasing or decreasing anxiety levels. And of course when you're working on conquering your fears, you certainly want to avoid exacerbating anxiety and panic! Nutrition is also exceptionally important when it comes to supporting the intense release work you have engaged in throughout this book so far, especially in neutralizing those toxins and the effects of stress. Food can also support you generally by boosting your energy levels and immune system so you are healthy enough in both mind and body to embrace everything that comes with breaking boundaries.

The term "comfort food" is pretty misleading; technically, the kind of food often referred to as such - calorific, high in sugar, fat and carbs, often fast or convenience foods - does not give any comfort when it comes to helping us feel anxiety-free. Instead it tends to lead to feelings of guilt, and physically speaking the excess carbohydrates and sugar leave us feeling tired and sluggish with brain fog. Certain foods can also cause, as well as exacerbate, anxiety through the chemical reactions they induce in the body. For example, anxiety can be triggered by increased levels of lactic acid in the blood.

Conversely, though, some foods are great at increasing levels in the brain of serotonin, a positive feel-good and calming chemical; others actually help reduce levels of adrenaline and cortisol (as discussed in Chapter Three, these are stress hormones that if over-produced are potent immune-system suppressors).

These hormones are also responsible for activating all the horrible symptoms of a panic attack like a racing pulse, increased perspiration, breathlessness, brain fog, involuntary shaking, feeling faint and dry mouth sensations.

Certain foods also contain powerful nutrients that can help counteract the effects of stress and anxiety that has built up over time, by keeping blood pressure within a good range as well as providing potent antioxidants to rid the body of harmful stress-inducing toxins.

It's also important to mention here that although you might not feel like eating before an event you are anxious about, lining your stomach will actually help to settle you and prevent your blood sugar level from crashing. If you avoid eating and your sugar levels do drop, your body will naturally produce adrenaline to push it back up, and this in turn will increase anxiety. Eating the right foods will also generate production of the calming chemical serotonin and tell your body that everything is normal and that it doesn't need to panic and use up your energy reserves because it doesn't know when it's next getting fed.

Foods to Avoid

- Caffeine
- Simple sugars (sweets/comfort/fast food)
- Alcohol

These three groups all increase blood lactic acid levels or stimulate adrenaline. It has been observed that even just cutting out caffeine results, in some cases, in the elimination of symptoms altogether.[11]

Foods to Eat

As with anything when it comes to nutrition, balance is the key and a healthy mindset will always ensure this. Being mindful in general about what nutritious value any food is giving us is important because certain diets (especially Western diets) can be lacking in the vitamins and minerals that are needed for optimal health, including psychological health.

In particular a correct level of the B vitamins is related to much better psychological health;[12] this may be partly because they contribute to helping you to feel more energized so you can work on losing any inhibitions and negative emotions that may have been preventing you from breaking your boundaries and pushing out of your comfort zone. Many factors can be responsible for depleting the body's levels of B vitamins, including sugary, white-flour-based, high-carbohydrate diets, perpetual stress and certain medical conditions, discussed in the next section.

Interestingly, in my own experience in practice a deficiency in B vitamins is often present in clients struggling with agoraphobia or worries about enclosed public locations or crowded areas.

This can similarly hold true for other anxiety-related conditions. A lack of B vitamins triggers signs such as stress and anxiety, uneasiness, irritation, fatigue and mental illness.

It's therefore crucial to include the foods below in your diet.

It can also be useful to add in a good B-complex multivitamin, especially if your general diet is lacking in the foods listed here.

Foods Rich in B Vitamins

- Leafy greens
- Whole grains and legumes
- Foods high in calcium and magnesium
- Seaweeds
- Milk
- Dairy products
- Sesame

Aside from the B vitamins, there are plenty of other important foods that help to counter the effects of fear and encourage better health due to their specific nutritional content.

Magnesium helps to regulate levels of cortisol (the stress hormone), so eat plenty of magnesium-containing foods:

- Spinach
- Broccoli
- Salmon and halibut
- Flaxseeds
- Sesame and pumpkin seeds

Slow-releasing carbohydrates (good sugars) help increase serotonin levels:

- Porridge
- Wholegrain cereals and bread
- Oats and barley (these can help to stabilize blood sugar and regulate moods too)

It can also help to have some wholegrain toast before bedtime to boost serotonin and help you sleep better.

Drinking warm milk before bed can also aid a better night's sleep; researchers have found that calcium can reduce muscle spasms and soothe tension, as well as reducing hormonal anxiety and mood swings. Milk also contains tryptophan and melatonin, two naturally occurring substances that help aid sleep and reduce anxiety.

Warm soya milk is useful if you are vegan or lactose intolerant as it also contains tryptophan, which is a precursor to the sleep-inducing compounds serotonin and melatonin. You can also get soya milk with added calcium to generate the same benefits as those provided by dairy milk.

Grapefruit, oranges, lemons and other citrus fruits are great for their high vitamin C content. Studies often show that very stressed people are deficient in vitamin C; it also helps to fight toxins released by stress.

Oily fish like fresh salmon and tuna contains omega-3 fatty acids, which are essential for the normal functioning of the brain. Most nutritional guidelines recommend having oily fish twice a week. Note though that due to the high temperatures used in the tinning process, which damage the omega-3 fats, tinned salmon and tuna don't count.

Black teas like breakfast tea and Earl Grey contain a natural substance called L-theanine, which has been shown in studies to create a relaxed yet alert psychological feeling. It also helps to negate the effects of the tea's caffeine (an anxiety stimulant). Plus, we're all familiar with the calming "have a nice cup of tea" effect! Be aware that adding milk or milk alternatives reduces the efficacy of the L-theanine. Drink your tea without milk, if you can, for better effects.

Nuts have a range of health benefits. Pistachio nuts in particular are rich in potassium and so help to control blood pressure. Research has shown that eating a handful every day can help manage cholesterol levels as well as reducing stress-associated rises in blood pressure.

Almonds also make a great snack as they are high in vitamin E to boost the immune system and B vitamins that help maintain the body's regular functions and metabolizing of glucose, which can help build resilience against stress. Again, a lot of studies in this area are based on consuming a handful per day.

Avocados also help to reduce high blood pressure. They can also be a great healthy alternative if you're craving high-fat food; try guacamole as a delicious snack or an accompaniment to most main meals like fish or chicken dishes, or as a tasty salad topping.

"Always laugh in the face of fear."

Summary

- Fears can be psychological or physical; but there's a way to deal with them all.
- Anxiety is not always what it seems: from hyperalertness to medical mimics.
- The metaphysics of anxiety pertains to the very origins of its manifestation, in not trusting the process of life.
- Certain foods and nutrition in general make an enormous difference to anxiety levels.

CHAPTER SEVEN

DETERMINING DIRECTION

D eep down, most of us have an idea of what we want in life – these are our deep-seated expectations, be they on a conscious, subconscious or totally unconscious (out of our awareness) level. The challenge comes, however, when we aren't always matching this in our current life, or for whatever reason lose sight of it.

This is often the point when people lose themselves, have breakdowns, experience depression, midlife crisis and so forth; because, whether they are consciously aware of this at the time or not, they are not meeting their true expectations, or aren't where they really think they should be in life in line with their core blueprint. This subsequently exacerbates their feelings of being unfocused, unmotivated or just distracted by life itself, such that goals, dreams and ambitions can be – and, sadly, indeed are – lost for many people.

One of the keys to avoiding all this is to know exactly what we want, understanding what's really important to us as individuals, who we really are and if we're matching it or not. Are we consumed by what we think we "should" be or do we really want to achieve these things? And do we need to break out and be fearless in changing any preconceived ideas and becoming someone new, with new ambitions – essentially breaking the mould to create a far better version of us?

Whatever your specific ultimate end goal, purpose and intention might be, and whether it's big or small, really doesn't matter. The purpose of this book is to enable anyone who so wishes to be equipped with the right resources to step outside their comfort zone to achieve anything they want to do. The point being that, once we're equipped with a strong sense of self-awareness coupled with the ability to deal with fear and limitations, anything is possible!

One of the most common things blocking people striving to get what they want is the fear of change, the fear of stepping outside their existing comfort zone and entering the unknown. However, the point of this chapter and Chapter Eight is to make this so much easier; to make the unknown exciting yet familiar territory that will become firmly imprinted in your neurology, such that any fear of the unknown turns into an exciting anticipation for the predetermined.

Getting What You Want

"I always knew I was going to be rich, I don't think I ever doubted it for a minute."

Warren Buffett

If you think about it, the people who know exactly what they want from the very outset and commit to that decision always seem to get exactly what they want sooner or later, in one way or another. Often, you can spot this in people, because they have an incredibly strong determination engrained in them, and everything is channelled toward it.

A great example of this is Warren Buffett, American business magnate, investor and philanthropist. Warren serves as the chairman and CEO of Berkshire Hathaway and is considered one of the most successful investors in the world with a net worth of $87.5 billion as of February 2018. This makes him the third wealthiest person in the United States and in the world. His statement, quoted above, encapsulates what I mean by strong determination and commitment to a decision.

Personally, I can confidently say that if I've ever *really* wanted something in life, I've got it. However, at times when I have found myself distracted, not wholly happy about something or slightly off course in life, I haven't achieved what I want. Rather I have just acquired a heap of challenges that have steered me in a different direction.

What's interesting about this is that if I've ever *thought* I wanted something but didn't deep-down want it, or if I didn't truly believe I was worthy of it, I haven't got it either!

This tells us a lot about where our real drive and focus comes from and how knowing that makes all the difference to the results we get in life. Quite simply, we must wholeheartedly deep-down want something so that we have enough determination and motivation to go out there and get it. We must also develop the self-awareness to distinguish the difference that always makes the difference.

Some questions to get you thinking:

- What is your life blueprint?
- Is this truly your blueprint, or someone else's for you?
- Are you living this?
- If not, do you still want this?
- Are you doing everything you can to achieve it?
- Have your blueprint and expectations changed throughout life?
- Are you on a different path from this now?
- Have you had the courage to admit this to yourself and taken action towards it?
- If money were no obstacle, meaning you could do anything – what would you do?
- What's really stopping you from doing what you want to do? (what's behind the surface reason .. and behind that . . . that will give you the real answer)
- What has to happen for you to achieve your goals? And what else? And what else? and keeping asking "what else and how" until you get to the answers you need.

Now are you brave enough with the belief, guts and determination to go out there and get it? To fully utilize all your talents, mind and creativity? This is the difference that makes the difference.

Determining and Driving Direction

Below are some keys to aid with real change and a checklist to help you determine a strong direction and highlight why certain things may not always necessarily be the best direction for you or how they could be blocking your progress.

Keys to Real Change

- Enjoying what you do and knowing for what purpose and intention you are doing it.
- Being consistent and in harmony with yourself about it, aligning all your life values to meet with your primary intention.

In other words:

- Does everything match to support what you want to achieve, or are there any blockages in the process making things harder for you or actually stopping you?
- If you're endlessly chasing your tail why is this so? You need to consider this on a deeper level.

Now is the time to dig in order to uncover any root blockages and resolve them. You'll only then find that your life aligns to support you and steer you in the best direction.

The checklist below will help you to determine if you have this in place. It can also be useful to get some external feedback by talking it through with a friend, so it's well worth considering the two points below.

- How aware have you made others of your intentions?
- Have you made yourself accountable yet? This will encourage that additional drive that comes from other people knowing.

The Checklist

Behaviour
- Do you do something every day toward what you want?
- Are you taking every opportunity possible?
- Are you actively making changes?
- Do you think and talk about this regularly, in a positive context?

What kind of language do you use?

- Are you going to "try" to do something, "hoping" something happens? OR
- Are you in the process of actually "doing" something?

The latter being the language you need to be using if you really believe in what you're doing.

Alternatively, do you seldom give it much thought, not have time for it, rather just expect it to happen – a bit like having a wonderful website and just expecting lots of visitors without somehow directing them?

The key is to always make sure your behaviour aligns with what you really want. If opportunities to help with this aren't presenting themselves, ask yourself why and whether this is what you really want.

Change is as powerful as it is scary, so you must really want something and behave as if you WILL get it, doing exactly what that takes, for it to become a reality.

Don't have dreams, have expectations!

Personality

- Who are you and who do you want to grow into?
- What traits do you need to exhibit to achieve the things you want?
- Does this align with your current personality?

Good external feedback from a trusted friend could be useful here!

There are plenty of resources throughout this chapter and Chapter Eight that will help you to better understand your own personality, and how this aligns with what you might think you want. This is a fundamental part of acquiring and developing the self-awareness to understand who you are and best determine your direction.

Enhanced self-awareness also reveals exactly why you may come across certain challenges or blockages in the process of achieving what you ultimately want, even if you're consciously and outwardly doing everything right and feeling that all is aligned.

Environment

- Are you surrounding yourself with the right people and putting yourself in the right places?
- Do you find you get support, encouragement and inspiration from those around you to support your outcome? Or
- Do you find yourself dragged down, left feeling uninspired with your spirits dampened by your surroundings?
- Do you ever seem to coincidentally meet people who just happen to turn out to be a great help with what you are doing and striving for? If not, question why not – what do you need to change?
- If you are working toward a common goal with someone, are they the right person/people to help you move forward? Are they aligned, or do they block progress, be this consciously or (most likely) unconsciously?
- Are they not as aligned and committed as they need to be and why?
- What might you need to do about it for the best?

This last point is a very important one because, as mentioned before, negativity breeds like wildfire and seriously affects progress and motivation. An analogy is lots of crabs collected in a bucket: they are mostly just crawling on top of one another, but there is one that's making a concerted effort to break free and is successfully crawling up the bucket to get out; however, all the other crabs keep pulling it back down – hence slowing the "freedom crab's" progress and mission by using up its energy and dampening its motivation.

Imagine if instead all the other crabs helped to push it upwards.

Our own environments are no different. Is yours in line with all the above and your end outcome?

Practicalities
- Do your skills, knowledge and talents align with what you want to do?
- Do you believe they are good enough to enable you to put yourself out there? Or
- Could this be a factor that is subconsciously holding you back?
- Do they meet with the criteria to make achieving what you want to do realistic?

This is a crucial element because often we have to further develop our skills and resources before we can fully move forward. When we are truly ready (and if all else is aligned) change tends to happen in a big way, and most often when it's least expected; so it's important to be properly prepared and equipped in a practical way.

Beliefs and Values

As you already know and will have imprinted on your brain once you've finished reading this book, beliefs and values are the most important aspect of anything you ever want to achieve. Because without true core belief, and if you are not doing something that is dear to you in terms of your values, everything else is futile; you won't have the true drive and motivation to achieve what you want.

You need to have a very strong positive purpose and intention for doing something to take you forward. This is what forms your blueprint; it is encoded deep in your DNA and your entire neurology – and not just meta-phorically speaking either!

Reading the rest of this chapter will help you to determine whether you are truly and absolutely aligned with your ultimate outcome, or if perhaps you need to change things.

The Right State

Whenever and whatever a situation may be, being in the right state will always help. Have you ever experienced something that has seriously annoyed, distracted or demotivated you and which has then made it exceptionally challenging to quickly and positively refocus because your mind is still in a negative state? If you have, you'll know exactly how unhelpful it is.

There was an occasion when, moments before I was due to leave the house for a local BBC radio interview, there was a knock on the door and it turned out to be a debt collector demanding a substantial amount of money for a supposed unpaid parking fine. There was no evidence to show why I was supposed to pay, so you can no doubt imagine how utterly annoying this was, not to mention distracting when I was focused on thinking about my interview. However, I was able to sort things out and on the way to the studio I utilized a good sense of humour and plenty of perspective on the situation to quickly change my state back to a positive, upbeat one, which allowed me to think clearly and do the best interview I could.

Children are especially good at instantly changing their state. When they've been told off for something, the petulance, tears or temper tantrums go on for just a short while and then they are soon laughing about something else, and it's all forgotten. Generally, this is because the child's attention and focus have been redirected (either by themselves or by an adult) to something else of greater significance to them such that it overrides the old state. As adults we can observe and learn from this how to change our state to a positive one to perform at our best and positively progress our outcome.

Ways to instantly change your state

Below is a reminder of some helpful techniques; they are described in more detail in Chapters Four and Six in "Anxiety-Busting" and "Reframing."

• Redirect your attention.

Focus on something that far supersedes the distraction:
What is more important to you?
What is your higher purpose?

- Separate intention from behaviour.

Look at why someone is doing what they are doing or behaving in an undesirable way, as opposed to what they are doing. It can help to understand them, calm the situation and even find a solution – remember the demanding boss and shoplifting examples?

- Create a resource anchor – your unstoppable emotional state.

This involves remembering a time when you felt unstoppable, superconfident, excited, fearless and carefree, as if you could do anything in the world. If you've never experienced that, imagine instead feeling this at a time in the future and use all your senses to associate into it.

- Have a sense of humour.

Think of something that always makes you laugh – a scene from a film or sitcom, something that happened to you that meant you could hardly control yourself for laughing or were bursting at the seams trying to remain serious. Alternatively, take the proverbial, out of yourself or a willing other; imitate people or situations to lighten things up and help you to see them differently.

- Peripheral vision and breathing techniques (in Chapter Four).

These are excellent in any context, be it in sports (particularly when taking penalties!), studying or work that you have to concentrate on, or any situation in which you need to control your state, feel calm and focus.

- Put it into a general perspective.

Is it really that important?
Is it anything you can't sort out or deal with?
Again, what's more important in the grand scheme of life?

- Have your own "Power Phrase" that triggers a feeling in you to stop caring, put things into perspective and move on.

It might be something that rhymes with "bucket" (!) or "Onwards and upwards", "Screw it, just do it", "Don't let the bastards grind you down", "Go for it", "Get outta my way", "Thanks for that" . . . whatever works for you.

Making Your Life GREAT™

GREAT is a simple mnemonic I developed after researching the key commonalities people had whenever they had successfully reversed a health condition in the gravest of situations; often when they had been given a terminal or life-debilitating and progressive diagnosis. I soon realized that actually, these are all key attributes of anyone who has achieved, or is in the process of achieving, immense success in getting their desired outcome in other contexts too.

It seems to me significant that the points involved in this could be organized into "GREAT", such a very appropriate word – because if you apply the following with full conviction, things really will be!

All the elements discussed in GREAT, and how to fully apply them, are also specifically referred to further on in this chapter as well as generally referenced throughout this book.

G Goals & Outcome
Establish clear, specific and determined goals

Anyone who achieves the things they want, big or small, has a goal and knows precisely their outcome; without a goal and an outcome we're simply drifting and existing. We can then create nothing to strive for or keep us motivated, challenged and excited, so we subsequently may not make the most of life and end up missing out.

In line with Locke and Latham's classic goal theory[13] and other research in the field of psychology, we know there is a clear relationship between goal-setting and improved performance. It is also the case that having very specific goals, as opposed to vague or abstract ones, make all the difference in attainment.

All successes start with a goal, but to turn these goals into a real outcome they need to be clearly defined, measured and driven by a strong motivation, intention and purpose. You can read more specific pointers on this later on.

R Responsibility
Personal responsibility NOT reasons

Consistently, with all great mindsets, comes an enormous sense of natural personal responsibility – "What's my part to play in this" thinking.

This means accepting responsibility for helping yourself. Always looking at what you can do to help the situation; and what and how you need to change and improve your life, as opposed to putting the blame elsewhere or relying on others or assuming it is they who need to change.

This is about taking personal control, because whatever else is happening in life, the one thing you can control is your mindset and your own reality and perception. This is connected to seeing the positives in something rather than letting the negatives automatically jump out – see the reframing material in Chapters Four and Six.

It's about deciding to take control and creating positive change rather than feeling like a victim or martyr.

This way, the change begins to happen and the more desirable results start to emerge on many levels.

E Emotional Well-being and Ever-Positive, Humorous Mindset

This is probably one of the most important factors because without both emotional well-being and a positive mindset, the rest is unlikely to materialize, or at least not in as profound or optimal a way as it otherwise could.

We all know negative emotion is the cause of limitations, blocked energy and manifested health conditions. So, the ability to positively and proactively deal with emotional challenges for heightened well-being is essential to all success in any context.

Mutually dependent on and connected to this is maintaining a positive mindset, always looking at:

What you can do: being a problem-solver and having a sense of humour along the way – the latter is an attribute always to be found in those who have achieved the major successes they wanted.

A positive mindset also includes displaying gratitude for all the resources and capabilities you do have and being appreciative of all experiences for the positive learnings they have provided to help you on your journey. Utilize your gratitude rock here, if you're using one. Touch it every time you are grateful for something and this will add to your positive "anchor" in addition to aiding a positive law of attraction to attract more of those things into your life. Chapter Eight, particularly "Entering The Quantum", will explore this further.

Appreciate the challenges and the opportunities that arise from them. There's always something positive to discover, whatever your sentiments may be at the time.

A Awareness and Absence of Panic

Develop heightened self-awareness and avoid panic when your path isn't seeming to go to plan.

In line with any success is heightened self-awareness to know when and what to change, recognizing in yourself when energy needs unblocking and the subsequent changes you might need to make. There is more on increasing self-awareness in this chapter as well as in Chapters Eight and Nine. A heightened self-awareness will allow you to discover how you need to best develop and tap further into your intuition for greater results all round.

It's also extremely important to be able, when things don't go according to plan, to avoid panic and the subsequent negative emotions that accompany it. And to appreciate that you will always face challenges for a reason and that it comes down to trusting in yourself and the process that you will overcome them – how strong is your belief? This too goes hand-in-hand with heightened self-awareness because if you know your true, wholehearted blueprint, you will be able to trust yourself and the process to plough through those challenges by addressing the unconscious root and blockages, or taking the learnings and resources you need to push further forward.

T Total Unshakable Belief System

Absolutely any successful person having achieved their missions in life will always, 100 per cent, have had an unshakable, total belief in what they are doing and their outcome (remember Warren Buffett?).

This must come from the unconscious root level, such that it is in your DNA. If you have this, no matter what comes to challenge you in the process and for whatever reason, you will be undeterred and you will achieve.

So if you have any doubts, get to the origin and work out why.

Do you really believe in yourself?

Is it what you really want?

Is there just a blockage of energy causing doubts that you need to address and overcome?

This is critical because you become what you deep-down, wholeheartedly believe at the unconscious level. Remember this is the ultimate consistent factor in getting what you want. If you have a deep-down unshakable belief system and no doubts, you will do it and you will become it!

You can now use GREAT™ as an easy but highly effective reminder of how to be exactly that in any context you desire.

Other Elements in Determining Drive and Direction

There are two dangerous ends of the spectrum where goals and direction are concerned, and either one carries a risk of unsuccessful results.

Often people can be so driven and focused when it comes to achieving their goals that they get themselves uptight and consequently in knots about it and it becomes counterproductive. They ask "Why hasn't it happened yet" and think "I'm doing everything, yet everything is going wrong."

All of this leads to feelings of frustration, upset, demotivation, burnout and so on. Moreover, notice where such comments are then directing focus – it's not on what you "do" want!

Conversely, at the other end of the spectrum is being unable to form an outcome and goal at all because of trying to force it, trying to be creative and feeling that you must come up with something. All of this equally leads to feelings of anxiety and complete overwhelm, consequently resulting in despair at the sense of moving nowhere.

Aside from the reasons already stated for this, it ultimately comes down to the need to allow for natural time and trust in the process of life, because either of the above scenarios indicate not having fully developed that unshakable belief system and total congruency with plans and core blueprint. Quite simply, when you are "really" ready, the time will come.

Although having an outcome is crucial, getting everything else in place also plays a critical role in actualizing that outcome. Practise everything GREAT™ and let things be. Trust in the process of life and go with the path of least resistance by working a positive law of attraction: that is, focus your attention positively, both at your deepest core belief system and in general thinking, to attract more positivity back into your life without resistance, as will be explained in greater detail in Chapter Eight. It is when you have all these elements in place and take the time to breathe that things will happen for you and take shape when you least expect them to. As the great Sufi poet Hafiz has it,[14]

"The pitcher needs a still cup for divine alchemy to work."

So, if you have all the critical elements in place, you can trust nature to take its course. This takes practice, guts and a strong head but if you have everything GREAT™ in place; it can be done and it WILL happen.

Alternatively, if you think otherwise, seriously start to look at why. Go back to self-awareness and then personal responsibility, then followed by emotional well-being and positive mindset. The answers will be there when you are most ready to find them.

Whether we choose to make positive changes in one big step or take small steps up to it, another key is that we need to have the right motivation.

Although we might often think we aren't ready to confront something, it's also a lot to do with whether we are motivated enough.

As discussed earlier, to achieve anything in life we need a strong, prioritized motivation behind it. It must be important enough to us, or we simply won't be focused or inspired enough to take action and do anything about it.

In some cases, we may need to be seriously disturbed about something before we act. A common if extreme example is when people have to experience a serious health threat or crisis before they act and change their lifestyle.

Conversely, we might be already naturally focused on our intention, such as losing weight to be healthy, look trimmer for a wedding outfit or photo shoot, or run a marathon or charity sporting event.

The bottom line is: we need to be bothered enough by something and have a compelling reason to take positive action, and remain positively motivated to reach our goal and ultimate outcome.

For instance, if I had a goal to get physically super-fit, it would be a total waste of time, because although that might be nice, and I'd always benefit from toning up, it's just not important enough to me right now. I would have no compelling reason because my body mass index (BMI) and general health is fine and deep down I'm happy as I am. However, if I discovered through my research that extreme fitness was the last necessary part of the process to fully reverse Type 1 diabetes, I might well suddenly develop a motivation to get in peak physical shape; I might even decide to take part in the notorious IRONMAN triathlon!

One way to find out how motivated you truly are about something is to ask yourself the following question and write down the answers very quickly as they first come to you in list form:

What's most important to you about living?

Keep listing any more that come to you, adding numbers to the list here, until you begin repeating the same ones.

The order in which you write things down will reflect your inner order of importance; so things that come to mind first and that you put at the top of your list are most likely to be the most important to you. And they are what really counts, because they come from your unconscious mind – the goal-getter – rather than the conscious mind – the goal-setter – which is what you'll get when you've had time to think about it, rationalize and list what you think the order of importance should be. The order of the list will also reflect your values – and these are crucial because they ultimately provide your drivers and motivation to act.

So did the highest intention of your goal – happiness, freedom, fulfilment (or your representation of these) – come near or at the top of your list?

Is your goal intention important enough to you right now to keep you motivated and doing something about fully achieving it?

If it's a little lower down than you'd have hoped, and you'd like a bit more motivation, have a think about your higher intention and why you're doing what you're doing. What needs to change? What isn't compelling enough for you? Keep going; you will get there!

If you still have challenges with your motivation and values, think about seeing a good clinical hypnotherapist, NLP master practitioner or coach (refer to the Resources section for guidance).

If happiness, freedom, fulfilment or whatever is the result of you releasing your fear are high on your list already, you'll likely experience exceptional results if you apply all the resources throughout this book. Keep focused and go for it! As with everything, you'll naturally find your own new challenges will emerge in the process; it's the ability to buck your fears, step outside your comfort zone and overcome these when the real change is happening that will allow you to achieve your goals. As I've said, it will most likely happen when you least expect it to, so enjoy and appreciate the process along the way.

I can also say with full conviction that my own personal and professional experiences have involved plenty of challenges and bumps that I've had to overcome along the road to successfully achieve the right outcomes. Some even seem unimaginable as they are so remote from my situation now, and that's not something I say lightly. So, prepare yourself to start getting the things you want from life. Just make sure you really believe you deserve them and are ready to overcome everything it takes to get them. If you do not believe this yet, it means you have a limitation with a far deeper emotional root behind it; the resources in Chapter Six will support you to tackle these head-on.

Positive Supports to Keep Driving Your Direction

In terms of breaking down boundaries and choosing to step outside of our comfort zone, our decision-making ability is pretty vital. This is because if we fear making the wrong decisions or procrastinate for too long about their consequences, it can prevent us making any decisions at all, stopping us from making that leap forward into new territory. However, the minute we can feel confident and fearless about our decision-making process, we open up so many more windows of opportunity to push our boundaries further, because with every action, there's a reaction steering you in that direction.

On the surface, decision-making is simple; it's the act of choosing between two or more courses of action and it's something we do all day, every day. However, as we all know, simple doesn't necessarily mean easy!

The complications come in when we become consumed with over-thinking about making the right decision because of its various implications; and there may not always be a "best" decision among the available choices. So, we must do the best we possibly can with the resources and knowledge we have and go with it, trusting in our deep core blueprint that whether or not the decision transpires to be right, wrong or indifferent at the time; it is always right in the long run.

If you've ever seen the movie *Sliding Doors*, it's a lot like that. You will, in the end, reach the outcome that deep-down fits your blueprint. Making a "wrong" decision at the time just means you get to determine the route to getting there, for whatever unconscious reasons or learnings you need. All the in-between bits – the so called "bad" decisions – are just a part of the process for us to learn, collect resources from, appreciate and move on from.

If we work intelligently with our decisions when we can, at challenging times, step outside our comfort zone and question:

- What are we being taught by life?
- What do we need to learn from the experience?
- What new resources can we use to push us further forward?
- Has a challenge led us to meet someone who we wouldn't ordinarily have met; what do such people or things help with?
- How's it changed your perspective?
- Has it provided you with a story to tell? Have you always been destined to write a book . . . ?

There are many of these questions, and the answers will be different and personal to everyone, but there is always something that will be extremely revealing and helpful in terms of your unconscious thinking and path forward. For example, do you attract challenges and unconsciously make bad decisions because you unconsciously punish yourself for something deep-rooted? Do you perhaps deep-down feel you need to go through hardship or certain experiences before you fully deserve to get what you were always destined to get according to your blueprint anyway?

It's therefore key to really probe into this and see that no decision is ever really wrong for you; it's just in line with you creating your own reality and what needs to or must happen for you.

While this is the case overall, though, we can still ease our journey by making the best decisions possible to help us through the process.

- Even if your decisions mean you're unable to correct past mistakes, allow them to aid improved decision-making in the future by taking all the positive learnings from it.
- Decisions can be made using either intuition or reasoning; but a strong combination of both is the most beneficial.

Effective steps in fearless decision-making:

- Turn more complicated decisions into simpler steps. You can do this by looking at the bigger picture by asking for what purpose ultimately is the decision and what's your ultimate intention in making it. What's the overall point of doing what you do, and does the decision dovetail with that?
- List all possible solutions/options – get them down on paper and talk it through with trusted, balanced, unbiased people. Things can seem less complicated and daunting when you externalize and break them down.
- Set a timescale and a deadline by which decisions need to be made.
- Get all the pertinent information you need.
- Weigh up the risks involved in each option by analyzing all the consequences.
- Do a values check on yourself: what is most important to you about the issue and whether your decision aligns with this.
- Which course of action is most advantageous overall, for the greater good and purpose?
- Consider your intuition as well as the facts and logic, never ignoring your gut feeling (See Increasing Intuition in Chapter Eight).
- Whatever decision you make, do you believe you are doing the best you can whatever the outcome? If you can say you are doing something wholehearted with conviction, you've reached the best decision.When it comes to deciding direction, while there may be big decisions to make, doing so can be made simple but all the same effective; sometimes the smallest things trigger the answer you need.

Practical Solutions

Often it can be easy to look at someone who has achieved their outcome and even think that they are "lucky". However, we tend not to see the years of challenges, blood, sweat and often tears that have gone into reaching their achievement.

The only difference between yourself and such people is time, personal experiences and their sheer belief and mindset to overcome and get through their personal challenges.

Listing things can help us with belief and mindset as it encourages us to see the problem in other ways and find what we need to do to be proactive in solving it. It also helps to create extra space in our minds.

Make three columns on a piece of paper, one headed "Problems", one "Solution Options" and the third "Actions".

Write down under "Problems" all the problems that result in limitations for you.

Write under "Solution Options" all the possible ways to resolve and overcome them.

Write under "Action" all the action you have decided on from your solution options and give it a nice big tick when you've done it.

Although some ways of solving the problem may not be desirable or necessarily easy, they are nevertheless a practical aid in the right direction to begin resolving limitations that are creating blockages. This will then help to create the mental space and time needed in the future for when you're ready to focus on and release any related root causes.

This is your "solution action list". Work through it a bit at a time to avoid any overwhelm. Do what you can, when you can. Everything is a positive step forward, and you'll ultimately feel better for it. Tick off each problem once you've blitzed it too.

If you can carry out a little task every day that allows you to make progress in sorting out a problem, things will soon change in a big way, and it will also help you keep your attention in the right place. It's important to reward your progress too – it gives you incentives to keep going and keep motivated.

Challenges	Solution Options	Action
Raising Funds	Changing Mindset:	Decision to…
	Strongly visualizing and feeling that you already have everything you need – go into that space in your mind. Assume you already have the funds to work your quantum reality (there is more about this in Chapter Eight). Keep your focus positive on everything you DO want, and CAN do – be the problem-solver, not -creator.	
	Practical: Extra work/ saving/consolidation/family or family help – individually or collective contributions, even in return for shares/skills etc./ formal investment/Kickstarter campaigns/sell items/Citizens Advice government schemes/loan options/ overdrafts/remortgage/refinance/seek out a good financial advisor – there's always something you can do – all kinds of weird and wacky fundraising – get creative!	

You can also use the table below to help set your own practical challenges, involving any fear that may be preventing you from unblocking anything listed above:

Negative Experience	Manifested Fear	New Challenge	Intention
Poverty as a child – always hearing "That's too expensive"/ "We can't afford that"/"You can't have that"/"Tough – you can't just get what you want"/ "Money doesn't grow on trees"/ "Money is the root of all evil".	Never having enough money to fulfil my goal.	Seeing money differently, as just "currency" – an energy flow. See value and appreciate what goes into goods and services – give money lovingly and be happy and grateful for what value you are receiving and all you do have.	Successfully unblock the flow of money coming my way so I can do all I want to do.

Negative Experience	Manifested Fear	New Challenge	Intention
Humiliation in school assembly when made to do a reading.	Fear of public speaking.	Speak at local public/social event – business network, church reading, school talk, wedding etc.	Successfully enjoy speaking at public events.
		Book a presentation skills session or course.	

If you have full conviction in whatever you are doing, and really want something, you will find a way and begin to see challenges as opposed to problems or obstacles. Assume the role of solution strategist as opposed to problem analyst, and you will do it!

Regularly ask yourself upon waking:

"What's happening today for me to take even more steps closer to achieving my goal?"

Goals with Purpose

We looked earlier, as part of GREAT™, at the critical element of having strong goals to determine any successful outcome. Here are some simple pointers you can apply to develop a solid goal for a solid outcome.

- What is your motivation and for what purpose? Is this strong enough to ensure that you act?
- Take small daily steps toward your goal. Support this by making yourself accountable in some way by creating an external check: get someone to ask you what you've done every day, vow to send yourself an email every evening on what you've done; whatever will make you feel accountable and so keep you pushing forward.
- Apply the process of SMART goals to make your goal specific, measurable, attainable, relevant and time-bound, with the added elements described below.
- Have benchmarks along your journey and reward yourself accordingly for each success.
- Perform a clear, detailed and specific visualization of your successful outcome using all your senses (and see "Quantum Reality" in Chapter Eight).

You may already know about SMART goals. This is a simple mnemonic used to really clarify an outcome to ensure that goals become a reality.

If you use the SMART technique together with GREAT™, you'll experience the difference between goals that always remain goals and goals that you actualize and which have a profound outcome. Therefore this process really can help you to determine direction.

1. Shape the specifics.

I wrote in my record of achievement when I was only 14 years old that I was writing a book about diabetes. In practical terms I wasn't – I didn't have any specific plans for it and I had no idea as to why, only that it would be something positive! I just knew it was something I was going to do; and, obviously, sixteen years or so later I did exactly this without consciously planning it at all. This just goes to prove that, above all else, deep-seated core belief and blueprint is the key, and intuition is always to be trusted.

Interestingly, when it came to the specifics that I hadn't consciously known about as a teenager, I was guided to them naturally while I was writing the book and up to the point of having it published. And getting specific was an important element in successfully materializing it into an outcome. Knowing all the details made me very clear and precise with my book proposal, which, coupled with a firm core belief and my natural blueprint, meant that the first publishers I approached offered me a contract.

So, there's a lot to be said for having a precise knowledge of what your goal is and how you're going to achieve it. For example, avoid vague and general statements, like "I'm going to improve my health" or "I'm going to be successful" – or even "I'm going to write a book!" Think about what specifically you are going to improve. In what context will you be successful? How, specifically? What's your target? And for what purpose are you going to do this? What's your motivation?

2. Make it measurable.

- How will you know when you have successfully achieved your goal?
- What must happen for you to know that you have achieved this?
- What evidence do you need?
- How can you measure your success; what can you judge it on?
- How would someone else be able to tell the difference?
- What is the specific benchmark that means you have got what you want?

3. Imagine your goal AS IF it is true right now.
Get a feel for this and programme it into your mind now, so you really know your outcome. Use all your senses to do this.

- See what you can see when you have already achieved your goal.
- Hear what you can hear. Are you saying anything to yourself, such as, "Yes! I've done it!" or is someone else congratulating you or complimenting you?
- Now feel the emotions that you feel when you have achieved your goal. Are you happy, laughing, excited, overwhelmed, amazed . . . ?
- Are there any specific scents present? Are you in a specific place?
- Are there any specific tastes present? Are you having a drink or something to eat as a celebration?

Really make sure you use all your senses and make the scene as specific as possible, with as much detail and clarity as you can. You know scientifically how visualization works – so positively utilize the amazing neurology we all have!

4. Make sure you have reasonable, relevant and realistic steps.
- Think up plenty of alternatives, should you need them, to achieve your goal.
- Do you have the right resources and support you need to achieve your goal?
- Have you allowed for a sensible period to achieve this?
- Do you have the right motivation and mindset required?
- Is your focus and belief wholeheartedly there?
- Is it what you really want?
- Have you got other flexible options and ways to achieve your goal?
- What other information and resources can you access?
- What other support can you get, should any challenges arise?

5. Allow time, and avoid leaving it open-ended.
- All too often, we say we want to achieve something but we either don't allow the necessary time frame to do this, or it goes on and on, meaning that we never really commit to an outcome and something always remains in the future. For example, if I didn't have a deadline and precise outcome, I might be writing this book for the rest of my life!

- On that note: be realistic but also specific. Ask your unconscious mind very quickly exactly when you will achieve this – which month, date, year?
- This way you will certainly know your outcome and your mind will know exactly where to focus. Imagine this as if it is already happening. Be sure to live it in your mind.
- Never be afraid to commit to a date. Trust yourself and remember this is a process that means different parts of your goal will integrate at different times, and sometimes before you ever imagined or when you least expect it (consciously at least).
- In my case, and things are always different for everyone, in reversing diabetes, my unconscious mind saw me achieving my outcome when I fully released the emotional root rather than the total physical release. Be mindful that the timescale is always different for different people; however, also know that you can just trust your mind and go with it.

If you apply all the SMART steps thoroughly, you'll embed them into your neurology so that you become focused – and, as you know by now, where focus and attention go, energy and results certainly follow, which is exactly what you want! Remember also how our minds work and visualize your goal with clarity and detail. The part of our mind that runs and maintains our body is unable to distinguish between what is real and what is not real; therefore, knowing our outcome can be positively programmed and preset into our entire neurology to achieve the precise results we want. This is explored fully with a specific technique in Chapter Eight.

Creating a Vision Book or Collage Board – Get Creative!

Creating a vision board is also a great way to keep you focused in the right direction, on everything you really want. It will act as a constant reminder of why you are doing what you do now, providing a great motivational boost. Really get creative here!

Daily Visual Indulgence

Every day, take just a few moments to close your eyes and see and feel your new life – whatever it is, feel it right now.

Headline Thinking

If you were to make your mark and leave your legacy, what would the newspaper, TV headline, Internet banner be; what would the strapline be that people would say about you? When all is said and done, what would you like to be known for and seen as?

"Determine your real direction and go for it."

Summary

- When determining direction, challenges come when we only think we want something and subsequently don't match our true blueprint.
- There are several ways in which you can discover your path and whether it is right for you, and once you fully establish this, you will find getting everything you want a whole lot easier.
- Creating a vision book or collage board can provide a great way to positively focus your mind on everything you do want and provide an excellent reference when you need reminding.
- Headline thinking will particularly help you to consider your purpose and what is ultimately important to you.

CHAPTER EIGHT

REACHING ZONE ZERO AND DARING TO LET GO

Reaching zone zero takes some doing: you have to have pushed through all your personal comfort zones to get to this place. Also, it's one thing to push through our personal zones but what is the difference that makes the difference and allows us to really feel and act like a zone-zero personality?

Zone-zero personalities, as well as exhibiting all the attributes and mind-set discussed in Chapter Five, are on totally different levels of thinking. A different mentality; this is more than just goals – it is about fulfilling your life purpose and about what you "want" as opposed to what you "need" to do to move forward and get what you want from life.

The difference that makes the difference being:

- No irrational fears or subsequent limitations.
- A strong self-awareness – knowing yourself so well you can recognize your own projections, such that when they need to change, you can act upon this to continue to best evolve throughout life.

It's about daring to fully let go and having that unshakable belief in yourself, your positive law of attraction – everything that you've predetermined for yourself that subsequently allows for you to trust in the process of life working for you.

Knowing that you have a deep-down positive law of attraction comes with knowing yourself and having a higher consciousness, so that you can attune yourself to feel and know your likely path, confident in the knowledge that everything that happens during the process is happening for a greater purpose – for you to learn and thus move forward toward your life intention.

This then allows for you to know you can deal with everything you need to and therefore go with it in the best way possible.

Displaying a zone-zero personality doesn't mean you never feel upset, angry, frustrated, misunderstood or susceptible to your own challenges; however, it does mean that you know why and what is happening, is happening. This massively shortens your refractory period (the time in which you experience negative emotions and allow them to affect you physically).

The "Yes" Universe

The "Yes" universe falls in line with quantum physics and correlates with the thinking of anyone in zone zero. Essentially, with everything you wholeheartedly think and believe, the universe responds to you with a "yes", irrespective of whether this is positive or negative. Therefore most people unfortunately don't get what they want from life, for what are often very unconscious reasons. This is why I say one of the fundamental staples to success is a strong self-awareness, which is inextricably linked to zone-zero thinking.

From seeing many clients who aren't where they want to be in life, be this in the context of health, relationships or professionally, I have observed and learned that it ALWAYS comes down to a deep belief (the root) that they don't believe they really deserve things, for whatever reason. This may be very unconscious self-punishment; a "not good enough" belief; guilt – including survivor's guilt, greed, religious values like original sin and so on . . . often they are reasons people don't connect themselves to or have ever consciously thought about.

On this note, clients often say the right thing but are still believing something else. For example, when I draw this to their attention and tell them I'm not wholly convinced of an unshakable belief, they always protest and say "But I do feel I deserve it and I do believe it" – however, once we probe a little deeper beneath the surface and get to the exact root, they discover that actually, they didn't really believe it or believe they deserved it! But as soon as they do, we then start to see real change.

In this respect we all create our own personal weather system: create a storm and expect it to rain, create clear blue sky and expect the sun to shine through. So be careful what you deep-down wish for: these self-fulfilling prophecies can be bad as well as good.

People often dismiss quantum or meta levels of thinking, but I think this is simply because of extreme fear; it's outside most people's comfort zone:

- It can be a scary thing to know and admit when you need to change to positively change things.
- It can be daunting to comprehend the workings of the universe and principles of physics because it means accepting personal responsibility for the life you lead.

So zone zero has a lot to do with whatever you do deep-down believe and want; with the universe saying yes to that; and to your ability to comprehend, accept and act on this. It involves losing the fear and putting the law of attraction into practice, which is exceptionally powerful stuff to take on and to master and which does break boundaries!

However, whether or not you choose to accept the "yes universe" and the law of attraction, it is always at work nevertheless. You will just be working it either positively or negatively. If you consciously choose to work it positively, you will reach zone zero and undoubtedly live an exceptionally fulfilled life.

In any case, the universe will respond to what you predominantly allow yourself to think and feel, and you will subsequently attract more of it!

As I always say, this is one of the most powerful pieces of knowledge mankind can possess. It is exceptionally exciting to comprehend that if you have the right thinking you can realize your own power and potential. There are some further, fascinating and inspiring resources at the back of the book that are well worth watching and can truly change your life. These will also help in explaining the scientific principles behind the "law of attraction" and why you will attract more back to you of those things to which you give your true focus and attention.

Developing Self-Awareness

This is all about noticing how you feel from moment to moment and being able to work out why, subsequently learning your own triggers, what makes you tick and why. It involves recognizing when you don't feel quite right about something and being able to work out the why behind the why and get to the deep roots without being afraid to explore this. Then it involves looking to what you can do about it when you need to . . . which can mean you need to have no fear of asking for help from a therapist, or of taking necessary action even if it's daunting.

Self-awareness can be developed quickly and effectively simply by considering and taking notice of the following factors:

- Noticing the language you use.

Written or spoken, is it:

    - Friendly, positive, "can do" rather than "can't do"?
    - Is it solutions-focused?
    - Is it going toward what you or others want?
    - Is it helpful or is everything a problem or never good?
    - If everything's a problem, why?
    - What's your general tone like when you greet a person or answer the phone, or type an email?
    - Do you tend to smile much, frown, feel relaxed, have background anxiety a lot; do you displace your emotions by taking things out on others?
    - What's your general attitude like, and why?

- Gaining objective perspective.

It can be useful to imagine someone is shadowing you all day and think about how they would perceive you and why would this be.

- What can you learn about yourself from this?

Equally, as suggested previously in the 30-day resilience-builders, ask others what they honestly think of you.

In this way you can get an objective picture as well as your own subjective analysis.

- Engaging in introspective self-indicators.

It can further be useful to find out your personal meta-programs and values: essentially, how you are hard-wired in terms of your psychological preferences – how you perceive the world, how you naturally function and make decisions. This can help to explain to you why you do the things you do and a lot of your thinking styles. These aren't in any way right or wrong; they are simply what form who you are, and they can provide you with indications as to your personality type that can be very helpful to explain why you may sometimes feel conflicted about certain aspects of your life.

For example, if you are in a job where you are constantly around people and directly dealing with them, yet you're more of an introverted personality, you may have been feeling uneasy about your work for a long time but not necessarily known why. Investigating your meta-programs and values can help you to understand what's wrong at work and how to change it, and could lead, for example, to you looking at developing your professional life so you can gain a more suitable role or work environment.

Alternatively, you could be a person who needs regular change and gets more energy from being around groups of people in a social setting, yet you may be married to someone who is content with routine and likes to stay in and wind down. If you've been unaware of the whys and of what makes both of you function best, it could explain some problems in the relationship you are in.

There are many online personality indicator tests you can take (and see the resource section at the back of this book for a very credible one). Do be aware that they vary in length and in what they really reveal. Having said that, simply partaking in them can intrinsically enhance self-awareness and understanding.

- Increasing your general awareness to increase your self-awareness.

General awareness as well as self-awareness is also key in terms of instigating change, simply because of how the mind and body are inextricably linked. All that we are aware of and let into our neurology through our five senses, everything we think and feel, affects how the body responds and the results we get.

How a Change in Awareness Creates Physical Change

In a study conducted at Harvard University,[15] testing whether the relationship between exercise and health is moderated by one's mindset, 84 female room attendants working in several different hotels were measured on physical health variables affected by exercise.

Those in the informed group were made aware that the work they do (cleaning hotel rooms) is "good" exercise and satisfies the recommendations for an active lifestyle. Conversely, subjects in the control group remained unaware of this.

Interestingly, although all other factors remained equal, four weeks later the aware group, who were now perceiving themselves to be getting significant exercise, showed a decrease in weight, blood pressure, body fat, waist-to-hip ratio and BMI; with the unaware group there was no change. This clearly supports the idea that when we have a greater awareness of something we physically respond to it.

So just think: with all the positive and proactive knowledge you have, both in general and about yourself, what positive results might you gain?

Expanding Your Understanding of the Mind–Body Connection

This is a great way to enhance self-awareness and deep roots. Although my first book *Mind Body Diabetes* is predominantly intended to help people with the condition, it's also a very useful general resource for understanding and exploring the mind–body connection. It introduces you to this topic and its vast proven scope. You can access the first few chapters freely on Amazon, or at www.dr-em.co.uk. You can access plenty of other free resources here too.

Applying all these factors will hugely help you to enhance your self-awareness, which in turn will always serve you well in living the best life you possibly can without the boundaries of fear and limitation.

Increasing Intuition

Intuition is about feelings, hunches and sensitivity, which all express emotion and sentiments without necessarily a rational explanation.

Quite simply, it represents our gut feeling. This feeling is hugely important because it is our unconscious mind at work – that is, the part of the mind that runs the body and keeps you safe, all of which you are not consciously aware of. Often it allows us to recognize or be alerted to something without us being necessarily sure why. We can learn to work with our intuition so feelings can be understood and addressed for the best outcome.

The ability to tune into our intuition and implicitly trust it is one of the most important life skills we can develop. It can sometimes feel like an almost overwhelmingly strong "call" to act, purely on a gut feeling rather than because of any conscious or concrete reasons.

A classic example is when you don't feel comfortable around a certain person; you have niggling doubts or there is something "off" that you just can't seem to put your finger on. There's no logical reason or anything factual to justify or explain the way you feel, but you do.

The reason for this is because there's something deep inside you detecting something amiss; perhaps it's from a deep buried memory and you're making subconscious links, learning from experience, or detecting something you don't even consciously know yet about that person, that's our intuition at play. For example, often when couples have been happily married for a very long time you hear them say "I just knew when we first met that we would get married." Such intense feelings come down to intuition; something deep in the minds of both individuals has linked the other person to something that gives them this assurance – perhaps they both have attributes the other has experienced before that connect with feeling loved and being safe or comfortable. Their minds may even sense a deep connecting synergy, or that some unknown amazing life event together is on the horizon.

In any case, positive or negative, our intuition is always designed to protect us, and whether or not it's always 100 per cent at the time, if you are in tune with your intuition and what you really expect from life at your deepest core level, it will be guiding you in the right way. Ultimately it will support you in line with all your other beliefs, thus providing the new learnings and resources necessary to move toward that. A good example being when I came to feel that the field of law as a career just wasn't for me; this was my intuition strongly leading me towards the path of what I do today, also aligning with when I was 10 years old and believed I would reverse diabetes, "knew" I would write a positive book about it when I was 14 years old and wanted to be a doctor in the field of helping people when I was only 4 years old. In any case, my intuition (despite it creating plenty of challenges at the time) ultimately led me to where I need to be, to align with my deepest core blueprint to be fulfilled.

The more we can all trust our intuition, the better, because it helps us to be more confident to make decisions, fully let go and trust ourselves to take the plunge and push our boundaries, stepping right outside our comfort zone.

However, because of the way we are often raised, and most of us having gone through standard education and work, as a society we are primed to do more left-brain thinking: to be concerned with logical, rational, hardcore evidence, facts and figures and so on. Logic of course has its place and must indeed be integrated – but too much left-brain thinking can limit our intuitive ability, and can lead people to question their intuition or others to ridicule it.

However, if we look carefully at the unconscious mind, it is clear that intuition accounts for all the digital left-brain information anyway. This information is all, once detected, stored in the unconscious mind, although we are generally not consciously aware of it for the simple fact that we'd have brain overload if we were! It's also worth knowing that when our unconscious and conscious mind aren't aligned, we can experience emotional turmoil and conflicting issues in our lives, which, aside from creating a miserable state of affairs, only presents us with more limitations that prevent us from pushing forward, breaking boundaries and experiencing the life we really want.

To paraphrase Dr Milton Erickson, a famous psychiatrist and clinical hypnotherapist renowned for his healing ability, "Patients are only ever patients because their conscious mind is out of rapport with their unconscious mind" Essentially, he means, when there's a conflict of deep-seated beliefs and the conscious mind is likely acting against your intuitive instincts that results in discord, manifested either psychologically or physically.

Increasing your understanding of your intuition can only help you in making decisions more easily and confidently and in being able to leap forward through and out of your comfort zone.

The evidence also lies in the fact that so many very successful people are also known to be very intuitive people; Richard Branson, the English entrepreneur and billionaire, is a prime example – he tells stories about his intuition in his books, describing intuitive business decisions or decisions made in his challenging adventures that have led to great success and to him saving his own life against the odds.

Being aware of exactly how intuitive you are will act as a good indicator as to how in tune you are with your unconscious mind and therefore how you can help yourself continue to push your boundaries.

On the next page is a quick intuition indicator, and, following that, ways in which you can work on increasing your intuition.

You find a series of 20 common statements that are consistent with intuitive tendencies; the more you find each premise resonates, the higher the level of intuition it indicates.

Remember – we're all intuitive, but to different degrees and in different ways; this exercise will assist you in recognizing which characteristics you exhibit most strongly and where you're personally at, so you can see how much it's possible to enhance your intuition.

You can take The Intuition Indicator™ online and receive your current intuition level instantly at:

https://intuitionindicator.questionpro.com/

Or take the test here.

The Intuition Indicators

Read the following statements and note for each one whether it is true for you – never, sometimes or always. For each answer give yourself a score of between 1 and 3 as follows:

Never = 1 point
Sometimes = 2 points
Always = 3 points

1. If you have a strong gut feeling, you'll go with this over logic, as it is most often right.
2. Upon meeting someone new, you instantly get strong positive or negative vibes, which are substantiated in the long run.
3. When you've been lost, you've successfully found your way back using your intuition.
4. You are extremely sensitive to feelings and often fully associate into (take on board/over-empathize with) the feelings of others, whether you want to or not.
5. You know your life purpose or mission in this world.
6. You don't mind going with the flow and spontaneity as opposed to rigid planning and routine.
7. Whenever you ignore a niggly gut feeling, you tend to find yourself later saying "I knew I should have trusted my instincts."
8. You've had vivid dreams, the events of which have then occurred in reality.
9. Your creativity is often inspired by your dreams and random ideas that just come to you and successfully transpire.
10. You often have periods of positive (excited/happy) or negative (anxious/sad) feelings before something good or bad occurs, without any explanation or actually knowing about something.
11. You often find yourself saying "I just know when I know" despite something being impossible to tell at the time; but it later turns out to be right.
12. You can feel when a loved one is hurting or someone you know has died, without prior knowledge of this.
13. You often make major decisions against the advice of authority or experts/family and friends based on what you've sensed or strong feelings, which always works best for you.

14. People often describe you as "creative".
15. People often joke that you must be "psychic".
16. You instinctively know when someone has a different motive and intention to what they are saying or doing.
17. You often just know or have a strong sense of what is wrong with someone before they say anything.
18. You've had foresight of a terror attack, natural disaster, crime, illness or death that later occurred.
19. If you have a big decision to make or feel unsure about something, you relax and meditate, trusting that the right answer will just come to you to make the right decision.
20. You can easily feel a strong sense of connection with people you've never met or places you've never been to.

Now add up all your points. Although most people score between 20 and 40, we can develop our intuition all the way up to 60. Naturally the more we are aware of ourselves and are open to exploring the power and capabilities of our own mind, the more intuitive we are likely to find ourselves being, and similarly we will be likely to feel more confident in pushing our own boundaries further.

Intuition Scores

Alert Radar (20–30)
This essentially indicates that you save and use your intuition for emergency situations; when you feel something is seriously not right and your life may be at risk. There will therefore likely be times when your intuition has caused you to act and has saved your life. For example, I remember when I was growing up and we were due to go on a family holiday to Cyprus, but my dad had a strange gut feeling about the holiday and changed the destination. As it turned out, the flight to Cyprus we would have been on sadly exploded on the runway!

While this amazing skill is obviously hugely important – obviously it can be the difference between life and death – it would be even better if you could trust your intuition enough so that you are never afraid to act on it.

To score above this bracket, you need to listen much more to your gut feelings, all those little niggles and hunches . . . Trust them and avoid being afraid to feel. We all have this capability if we allow it and explore it.

Emotional Radar (31–40)

Scoring between 31 and 40 indicates that you are particularly sensitive to the feelings of others and can develop very close connections with people. This includes understanding them, feeling their projected emotions and feeling for them. You'll probably often feel that you are on the same wavelength as those who you are close to, finding connections easy to make. You'll therefore tend to use your intuition to gauge the emotions of others.

Naturally this is a great ability to have when positively used for developing good relationships and helping others. However, intuition can extend so much further; try continuing to explore this, and apply it in a much wider context, perhaps in the areas where the life discovery model highlights (see later on in this chapter) would prove useful. You're clearly very capable of positively tuning in to your intuition and using it with great effect. On which note, enjoy exploring it to push your boundaries even further to see where it can take you by fully trusting your inner voice.

Guiding Radar (41–50)

With this score you'll tend to be a very intuitive person, and extremely aware of your emotions personally and your connection with the universe, which you'll know is exceptionally useful in a whole range of ways! You know how to use your intuition and trust it to drive you to where you need to go for the best outcome in any context and aspect of life, but particularly when it comes to being creative and moving forward overall.

Naturally the more you work with your intuition to enhance it, the more you'll learn to trust it, which you'll find will make an enormous difference to your life.

Hyper-intuitive Radar (51–60)

Congratulations! You have a fantastic skill that you've already tuned in to and trust, indicating you've more than likely scored high on the Zone Test as well.

Clearly you are able to consciously tap into both your unconscious and subconscious mind for the best results for you; and quite probably for others too. Irrespective of whether an outcome is good, bad or indifferent at the time, you implicitly trust your intuition to ultimately lead you down the right path for the right reasons, toward achieving your life mission and purpose.

You'll therefore already appreciate the benefits of working with your intuition; it's likely that you meditate regularly and are open to enhancing your intuition wherever possible, enjoying doing so and experiencing very powerful, profound, unlimited results.

The real question for you is how far you choose to utilize your intuition and enjoy exploring new boundaries, for unique discovery and higher purpose on a universal level.

Resources to Increase Intuition

The higher your intuition range according to this indicator, the more likely you are to push out of your comfort zone, because your intuition will always signal to you if you are safe to do so and whether you're doing the right thing or not. This doesn't mean you'll always make the right choices and decisions at the time; but they will always be right in the long run, for your ultimate purpose.

Whatever your intuition indicator result is, the next step is about looking at how you can best increase this fantastic natural resource by tapping further into your unconscious mind, heightening self-awareness and general consciousness and having the confidence to implicitly trust yourself and the process of life to support you in line with your core beliefs, blueprint and expectations.

- **Pay more attention to how you physically feel about something – and question exactly what this feeling is.**

Personally, when I feel extreme nervousness, about something, there's a big difference from when I'm just feeling "natural" nerves; this is how I know my unconscious mind is alerting me to something not being quite right.

I have also in the past been alerted physically when something was seriously amiss. On one occasion I had a very serious negative gut feeling and it led on to a severe physical reaction - it literally made me sick and very feverish (that's metaphysics for you; this situation did make me feel psychologically sick to my core and I was mentally and therefore physically reacting to this as the thought of it metaphorically made my blood boil and made me want to get it out of my system). Interestingly, and reassuringly, the subsequent turn of events (because of how ill I was), thankfully steered my partner and me in a safe direction, providing us with all we needed for the best outcome going forward.

Always notice if something is "bugging" you so much that it's making you feel ill, and question it – what is it all really about?

Notice your natural, instinctive emotional responses to things and, again, question this. For example:

- Have you randomly burst into tears for no seeming reason?
- Become suddenly snappy and angry about something but have no conscious idea why?
- Have you felt giggly about something when nothing was particularly funny?

Essentially, notice your emotions that are without rational explanation and question why this may be so.

- What's your unconscious mind trying to really tell you and alert you to?
- What really needs addressing?

This indicates that intuitively you are or aren't happy or feeling wholly right about something.

- **Add random things into your day or week whereby you can do something totally different and refreshing from your normal routine.**

This might only be a walk to the coffee shop, but if it allows you time to be in a different space, have a change of scenery and change your focus, acting as a positive distraction; it will help with creativity and making space in your mind, giving you a greater opportunity to hear your inner voice.

I'm sure you've experienced it before – you've been out walking, or in some new or random place, and you've come to a sudden realization or decision about something when you were least expecting it. This is exactly that: it's simply creating the space for things to come to you naturally. Intuitively, you'll detect this and receive the answers from your inner voice!

- **Consciously decide to trust yourself and get into the habit.**

This really is about letting go of inhibitions, fears, and limitations to trust yourself implicitly and get rid of the conscious clutter so you can turn your focus to the right decision for you. It's a little like if you've ever lost something in a room amidst a clutter of other things: you just can't seem to find it no matter how much you search; but eventually you do find it – typically when you're not actually looking for it.

So, although it might seem hard to find the answer sometimes, it's about trusting yourself to know it's there. It may be buried deep down, but if you trust yourself implicitly it will come to you.

- **Get into the right, calm state.**

Being in a calm state is key otherwise you won't be able to hear any inner voice or notice how you really feel. The resilience-builders, peripheral vision and breathing techniques in Chapter Four will help a great deal with this.

- **Utilize brainwave meditation.**

There are lots of different ways to meditate, and they all have fantastic benefits. The fundamental principle is to clear and declutter the mind, allowing for your intuition to be heightened and for you to be at your most receptive to communication from your unconscious mind.

The reason I suggest brainwave meditation here is because this is very specific in using binaural beat music, which actively lowers your brainwave activity, taking you from stressful states to useful calm and relaxed states in which the unconscious mind is scientifically proven to be most effective.

Alternatively, praying, listening to music, gardening, walking, colouring or pursuing arts and crafts can also act as forms of meditation depending on your own inner workings; of course, you'll know best, deep down, what works for you.

The ultimate aim is to become freed from your unhelpful conscious thoughts; if your mind is still and quiet, without conscious clutter, it will have the space and ability to allow much more of the right stuff to pour in and do its work. Think about shaking a cup around while simultaneously trying to pour water into it; you'll get far less water in than if it is held perfectly still!

The Practical before the Quantum

Before we step into the exciting quantum world of predetermining your destiny, it's critical to ensure you fully let go of and surrender your fears first, so there's nothing holding you back, either consciously or unconsciously.

It's also important to clarify and nail what you really want from life – to distinguish between what you might think you want and what you actually want deep down, and your ultimate purpose. This really does make a difference in terms of how easy your path will become.

Here is my own personal experience of the difference between what someone might think they want and what they really want in line with their true life blueprint:

From the age of 14 I was set on becoming a barrister, ever since a teacher and a few other authority figures including a county court judge had told me I'd be very good at it. I thought for a long time that this was what I really wanted, and I went through A levels, law school, work experience and so on.

But just about every curveball you might think of was thrown at me during this process, ranging from an undiagnosed rare genetic condition with serious symptoms and Type 1 diabetes consequently going awry to financial challenges, relationship and a whole host of other equally surprising issues. It was all driving me insane; at the time, I could make no sense of it.

I finally came to realize (or to admit to myself) that actually law wasn't the path for me and in fact conflicted with many of my deep values.

And after much self-analysis I realized that I only ever thought I wanted to be a barrister because I'd been told I would be good at it and subsequently encouraged in it. It dawned on me that, alone, I wouldn't have chosen this path; I'd always been more naturally interested in health, medicine, healing and helping others.

I eventually realized that I held a very deep unconscious belief as a result of being discouraged from science subjects at school. I needed to create real change around this, otherwise life was never going to fall in line with my true blueprint .

Eventually I decided to study what I really wanted to and, in what almost seems like the blink of an eye (albeit with its challenges), I had gained a doctorate in the subject and built up a successful practice; I'm an author in my field and I run training courses in the subject too.

It is vital – truly life-changing – to determine what we really want rather than what we think we want because of outside influence and/or our own limiting beliefs or conflicts.

The Life Discovery Model

This model can help you to look over all areas of your life and assist with highlighting incongruencies and conflicts.

There are so many components to our lives that it can be only too easy to miss aspects that need fulfilling or changing. Especially as sometimes these are aspects that we're consciously unaware of or have never paid much attention to. We can therefore have unconscious conflicts going on, shown to us only through our physical or psychological health and that we don't necessarily pick up on. However, when we do take the time to engage in a life audit of the kind this model is designed to guide us through, the results can be incredibly revealing and not only help align our long- and short-term aspirations, but also help us to discover our true meaning and purpose.

This model is based on looking at the five main areas of life – mental, emotional, physical, practical and spiritual – that shape who we are and how we feel. It provides a comparison between the current life you're experiencing and the intended life you want and would like to experience, so you can discover how these align, what they might reveal and what changes you might want to make; you will be able to see everything you really want and discover anything new that you didn't realize you wanted.

As you run through the model, the answers it gives will enable you to access how fulfilled or complete as an individual experiencing life you feel overall and, most importantly, what needs to happen for you to feel fully complete, and exactly how far you need to push yourself to embrace fulfilment for you.

For a quick indication of the areas of your life you most wish to develop and those you are currently content with, you can compare how many ticks (depicting happy) and how many triangles (depicting need for change) you have.

For instance, like in the example shown, in the "current" box write down your current situation relevant to the category listed on the left-hand side. If you are happy with this, place a tick in the right-hand column next to it. Conversely, if you are not happy with this, or would simply like to change things, place a triangle in the same column. In the "Aspiration & Action Toward" column, write down any new choices you would like to have a go at or achieve within the relevant life area stated on the left. Then write down all the things you can do to take action toward making these changes from your current situation to a more desirable one, for that more greatly fulfilled life.

Life Area: **Mental**	Current	Happy or Change	Aspiration & Action Toward
Occupation/ employment status	*Police officer*	▲	*Develop own business; Savings personal funds, biz plan, e-biz course*
Personal interests (current affairs, travel, fashion, business, anthropology, politics, food etc.)			
Personal & professional development (courses/reading/ research/excursions/ workshops etc.)			

Life Area: **Emotional**	Current	Happy or Change	Aspiration & Action Toward
Relationship (single, dating, married, partner divorced etc.)			
Family (close/ children/parents) Friends (good/close/lots/ supportive)			
Emotional support (who, what, how strong, any mentors)			
Emotional health (consistently content/ happy/ unhappy/ temperamental/ up and down/depressed/ stressed/confused etc.) Self-understanding and awareness (excellent/good/average/poor)			

Life Area: Physical	Current	Happy or Change	Aspiration & Action Toward
Physical health (excellent, good, average, conditions, illness) Regular activity/exercise			
Physical intimacy (happy, content, average, challenges, N/A)			

Life Area: Practical	Current	Happy or Change	Aspiration & Action Toward
Lifestyle (socializing/hobbies/ /smoking/drinking/diet/ holidays/breaks)			
Financial (income/personal transport/ home-owner/ debts/investments)			
Logistics (living arrangements/ location work, travel strains/you time)			

Life Area: Spiritual	Current	Happy or Change	Aspiration & Action Toward
Life philosophy (religion-driven, live and let live, liberal, N/A etc.) Personal contribution to life (what you've personally contributed so far to life – children, saved lives, books, employ, invent, teach, research etc.)			

Life Area: **Spiritual**	Current	Happy or Change	Aspiration & Action Toward
Higher life purpose – fulfilment for you (help, cure, entertain, innovate, inspire, lead, develop, etc.)			
Universal connection (utilize intuition, meditate, visualize, explore/research/ apply the law of attraction – quantum/metaphysical field)			

Now look back over the model as a whole to:

- Compare how many ticks and triangles you have.
- Look at which areas of life your results indicate you'd most like to change or develop.
- See in which sections you are most happy and where you find greater purpose and interest.

Then look over the "Action Toward" column and observe the following:

- What, if anything, is really holding you back from pushing forward with the action you have determined you need to take. This will help you uncover the root of the root if you keep asking why.

Now, taking the first figure that comes in to your mind up to 100, give yourself a percentage score of how complete you feel as a person right now:

Completeness Score: ☐ per cent

Critical Question: Now, looking at your model, what must happen for this score to reach its highest level possible? For example, if you gave yourself a completeness score of 76 per cent, what is that missing 24 per cent that has to happen in order for you to reach maximum fulfilment? Filling in the following table may help if you're unsure; the filled-in example will provide you with an idea of this.

- What do you ultimately feel you need to do, and for what purpose?
- What kind of things do you actually want to do?
- What are you driven by – causes, religion, self, family, pragmatism?

Do you find purpose in doing things for:

- Specific groups
- Social duty
- Family
- Causes or charity
- Individual intent
- A global greater good

Life category	What you haven't explored in life yet	What you'd like to explore
Travel	All continents	Sabbatical/gap year to travel around the world
Learning and education		
Culture		
Creative arts		
Theatre/drama/dance/writing/producing/film/music/art/design/performing/magic etc.)		
Fun/comedy (doing or watching)		
Healing, health, metaphysics		
Universal understanding and connection		
Quantum physics/meditation/spirituality etc.)		
Personal understanding of the self		
Work opportunities		
New hobbies and interests		
Adoption/fostering		
Starting or expanding a family (kids/pets!)		
Relationships/dating/sexual interests		
New careers/work opportunities(working with animals instead of people/different age groups/creative as opposed to digital/less pressure/fun/more responsibility/team work or individual etc.)		
Business/investment/mentoring/coaching/charity		

Do all these align with the things you want?

So once again here comes the critical question . . .

What action do you need to take for you to reach maximum completeness and fulfilment?

Now you can use all your answers to form an ultimate action list – a life list – of all the things you want or need to do to enjoy a fulfilled journey forward in life, with nothing to stop you.

Entering the Quantum – A No-Comfort-Zone Area

Having now gone some way through this book, worked on all your fears, limitations, inhibitions and knowing what it takes to fully let go and become a zone-zero personality, if you're not already there you'll be some way towards knowing exactly what you want from life, in any context.

We can now have some fun with the quantum and making this a reality.

When it comes to quantum physics, quantum reality or mind–body metaphysics (metaphysics being the very first principles of things, including abstract concepts such as being, health, knowing, identity, time and space), comprehending and applying it allows for no boundaries in thinking. It's certainly a 'no-comfort-zone area' and the following quote[16] sums it up brilliantly:

> "No development of modern science has had a more profound impact on human thinking than the advent of quantum theory. Wrenched out of centuries-old thought patterns, physicists of a generation ago found themselves compelled to embrace a new metaphysics. The distress which this reorientation caused continues to the present day. Basically, physicists have suffered a severe loss: their hold on reality."
>
> Brye DeWitt and Neill Graham

And now the brave can explore, enter and utilize a new, exciting reality . . .

Quantum Reality

There are many excellent books and other resources on this subject that you can explore if you wish to learn more in depth (and some are listed in the back of this book). It's a vast and fascinating subject well worth exploring.

For the purposes of this chapter, we're talking about quantum reality as opposed to the small proportion of reality that we perceive through our five senses of sight, sound, taste, smell and touch.

When we talk about quantum reality here we're referring to the basic core physical principle that like attracts like in terms of particles and energy.

Quantum reality is a place that exists beyond time and space as we know it; it's where the metaphysical (the intangible such as thoughts, beliefs and emotions) meets with the material realm to decide on a future outcome. The material world that we sense through our five senses only makes up a very small percentage of the whole structure of reality. Quantum physicists have discovered that a healthy human brain can process more than 400 billion bits of information per second. Out of those 400 billion bits of information, we are only consciously aware of about 2,000 bits.[17]

Looking at the big picture, this suggests that our conscious awareness of reality is minuscule - lower than 1 per cent - thus most of what we understand as reality is taking place beyond our five senses, and consists at least partly of the interactions we create between the material and intangible energy. Essentially, we are often determining our future through our deep belief system, thoughts and emotions (all the intangible elements that create energy and determine whether this is positive, indifferent or negative), without even being aware of doing so. This is what gives rise to the "law of attraction" - genuine positivity and an unshakable core belief in something attracts more of the same positive energy to it, and causes the universe to respond accordingly. Equally, as we've previously mentioned, the same applies in a negative context by way of continuing negative cycles.

Such revelations are exceptionally exciting when we are aware of the quantum: imagine what we can further derive from this; we can consciously determine ourselves through our deep inner belief system and thinking, what we subsequently do in and attract into our lives.

With this information we can take our goals one step further by embedding them into our future, truly making them a predetermined expectation.

Although we tend to think of a memory as something that happened in the past, in fact memory is just the process by which we encode, store and retrieve information that is outside our present world. So we can also have "future memories", or to put it another way, strong visions and deep inner core beliefs, that determine where we're heading.

Following are two small but fabulous examples of quantum physics and the law of attraction determining a positive outcome. They were both told to me by a client of mine, Jasmine; following the work she and I did on her case of "anxiety" (documented in Chapter Six), she was doing some advanced progressive work with me.

"I was on the bus on the way to meet my friends when it broke down in the remote countryside. The driver told us it was going to be two hours before a replacement bus would be able to reach us, but I thought to myself and believed "There's no way I'll be sat here for that long." Fifteen minutes into the wait, a family behind me tapped my shoulder and asked if I'd like to share their taxi! Of course I did – and incidentally had a great fun journey with them they were all going to a family party – they even invited me to join them for a drink. Out of all the seats I could have chosen to sit in, I had opted to sit in front of this family, so I was the one they invited to share the taxi with. Had I not been aware of this I really think I'd have had my usual old-style bad luck and not got a look-in. It's hard to believe but creating a positive law of attraction and the quantum world seriously works."

"I had been on a day out shopping with my friends and they noticed that I hadn't got one of my shopping bags with me. I retraced my steps to try to find where I'd left the bag, but to no avail. My friends were adamant that someone had walked off with it, professing that there were some terrible people about. However, I thought to myself "I WILL find it, I know someone will have handed it in."

At the end of the day we went our separate ways; but I was still determined on a different outcome, so I decided to go back to the store where I had been shopping – and this time, someone had handed in my bag! So despite the odds, my thinking, deep belief and therefore my decision to go back again led to another positive outcome. The old me might well have just listened to my friends, felt disappointed and left it."

It can be easy to put this kind of thing down to coincidence; but we all still create those "coincidences" through what we either consciously or unwittingly put out there to the universe via our thinking and deep belief system. Remember "like attracts like" at a core level; so once you choose to positively work this, your life will change beyond recognition.

Although we are unable to control other people's law of attraction and what they put out there in line with their personal deep beliefs, we can control our interactions with them, how we respond, where this leads us and what it determines.

So, from the small to the almost incomprehensibly huge, we can determine our "future memories" and a positive law of attraction for ourselves when we understand the science behind it and adopt the right thinking, belief system and positive core.

It's Written In the Stars

This is a familiar expression. This section explores, essentially, the science behind it, and provides us with the tools to create our own inscription in the stars.

By this point in the book you have worked with ensuring that you have no conscious or unconscious blockages of energy and that you know exactly what you ultimately and really want and believe at your deepest core level.

Things that are "written in the stars" or were "always going to happen" for anyone are only so because people have always had such a strong belief and natural inclination toward something that they have unconsciously determined it.

Quite simply, we all have something "written in the stars" or that was "always going to happen" because we all have our unconscious beliefs and blueprint; however, many people let this be obscured or blocked by negative deep-down limiting beliefs and values. Thinking and beliefs along the lines of "Things like that don't happen to me" previously discussed, especially in the context of the "Yes" universe.

However, the great news is that with a strong self-awareness and having worked through this book, you can go for what you want and begin experiencing the positive changes that will subsequently start to occur in your life to support you in your journey toward this.

How to Create Your Future Reality Using the Quantum

You can also access this process freely on audio, including music, under audio resources on my website.

The Installation Process

1. Know your intention for doing and achieving what you want to and make this your focus.
2. Imagine you are already living this reality – just as you did with the SMART goals in Chapter Seven.

Imagine the last step that must happen for you to know you have successfully achieved this. How do you know it's a reality?

See clearly what you can see with as much detail as possible – who or what is there? Where are you? What are you wearing? What else can you see around you? What do you look like? notice how different you look.

Hear what you can hear – are there any noises? Is anyone saying anything to you? Are you saying something to yourself?

The crucial factor – "feel" the change! Associate so heavily into this that your entire body is consumed with it – let every one of your cells feel it.

Really enjoy feeling this shift. Observe: are you displaying your emotions physically or externally in some way?

- What scents do you smell?
- What tastes do you taste?

Use all your available senses to make this experience as prominent, real, detailed and clear as possible. This is your reality. Create a permanent space in your head for this so it is a place you can visit daily. Take note: this takes practice and focus; you can't just think it once and have it come true!

3.   Now put on some brainwave music, preferably gamma wave music.

I find "Brain Massage" or "Brain Power" by Kelly Howell from brainsync.com work well. Remember to use headphones for the best use of brainwave technology too.

4.   Now spend 20–30 minutes fully and only associated into your future reality . . . See what you can see, hear what you can hear, feel the deep core feelings you can feel, take in all the scents and tastes around you.

Throughout this experience, really allow yourself to let go and feel the shift and the change in your cells, in your gut – feel the difference.

5.   During this time, make a decision.

Decide to change, from your old existing personality with its limitations and fears to the new fearless you before you allow yourself to leave your meditation.

6.   Now step out of this experience.

Imagine you are looking at the experience as if it is a photograph you are holding in your hand. Look at this photograph with excitement and joy as something that has already happened. Keep focused on those associated feelings, take three long, deep breaths (in through your nose and out through your mouth) and feel a positive surge of energy rush through you, down your arms and into the photo of this future memory. Keep hold of this positively charged picture.

7.   Prepare to travel into your future.

Now, still holding this energized photograph, close your eyes and imagine drifting out towards your future.

8. Stop, and hover above where you feel is the right time and place.

Avoid forcing this and go with what your mind presents naturally to you. If this is really in your deep belief system, you can trust your mind will know the right time and place this is to occur. Now gently drop your photographed future memory down into this part of your future life. See it float down and click in perfectly. As you do this, hear it lock into place, as it now becomes firmly locked into your future. As you do this, hear the sound of a lock or a door shutting.

9. Travel back to the present.

Once you've done this, as you begin drifting back toward your present life, notice how when you glance down, everything else in your life adjusts and aligns accordingly, in order to support you in having successfully already achieved this future memory. And know that everything that happens from now on is always happening for a reason (whether at the time it feels good, challenging or indifferent) to support your ultimate outcome becoming a reality.

10. Drift back into your present body and enjoy!

Remember to keep visiting and feeling your quantum reality in your mind. Feel the changes and embrace the new decisions you've made. Enjoy and get used to the new fearless personality you've created.

Again, revisit feeling your reality as regularly as you can, apply the necessary changes to be the new you and create those changes, making that decision at your deepest core level. Remember that the only reality in your life is your own reality – everything that you play out in your head and choose to be!

Your outcome is now heavily imprinted in your entire neurology through every one of your senses and cells. You have an indestanding of how the mind–body connection works as it has been discussed earlier in the book, along with the workings of the universe beyond pure material physics; so you know there's a lot to be excited about!

I've done this type of work with many people, myself included, and I've always known it to work when done properly with full conviction. Although some people might find this technique a little out there – it does push some conventional beliefs and thought boundaries – it will seem more acceptable the more you can appreciate the science and workings of our neurology and the universe, and of course the more you have moved out of your comfort zone!

Anyone who wants to can and will experience phenomenal results, but it all has to start with the right mindset and adapting yourself to fully transition and make the necessary changes to be the personality who has everything you want. Become your reality and feel that your ultimate outcome, intention and higher purpose are happening now.

> *"The universe is always listening, and quantum physics is at play – good, bad or indifferent."*

Summary

- Reaching zone zero is about fully letting go of irrational fears and limitations; developing a personality where you enjoy breaking boundaries, fully understanding yourself and knowing your purpose, always seeking to fulfil it.
- A large part of reaching zone zero is fully appreciating the workings of the universe, recognizing the "Yes" universe and making this work for you, too.
- It is also about self-discovery and developing a higher consciousness to understand yourself and others, so you can positively adapt and change when necessary or make the most of everything.
- An appreciation of quantum and metaphysics will greatly assist in this, along with introspective questioning and understanding, enhancing intuition, carefully going through and applying the life discovery model and daring to practically enter the quantum.

CHAPTER NINE

RETAKING THE ZONE TEST

You have your zone score from Chapter One that enabled you to see just how far you were likely to step outside of your comfort zone and break the kind of boundaries that really make a positive difference to your life.

Now, having read this far in the book and applied any relevant work to help you push your own personal boundaries, you can go back to Chapter One (or take it online, as before) and retake the test to see just how much change you've implemented, as well as highlight any points you may still identify and wish to address to keep moving forward, getting to where you want to be and enjoying a full life beyond limits as a zone-zero personality.

In retaking the test it's important to remember this is a measurement tool for you and your own personal development in whatever area you wish; so you'll get the most out of it if you again answer the questions as honestly and quickly as possible. If your score isn't as expected, keep rereading and applying all the resources in the book; you will get there.

Zone Test Scores

The Comfy Zone (<50)

You still like your comfort zone. This is great if you are genuinely happy and content where you are right now. However, if you're not, in any area of life, then it's time to make that decision and use this book to really break free and make the most of everything you can. You've undoubtedly heard the expression "Life's too short"; it is somewhat overused and may have slightly lost its meaning but it really is true, and there's so much out there to be explored and enjoyed. Never fear yourself – and if you have any doubts, the following chapter may contain a few words of inspiration. In a nutshell, enjoy your existence in the best way for you, knowing that whatever the situation, you always have choices.

The Exploring Zone (51–74)

You are warming up for action and you have a lot of exciting things ahead of you. You now know the kind of things you need to do and work on, so it's a case of turning any nerves and limitations into excitement and energy for all you'd like to be and achieve. Work on your confidence and letting go of everything that may be niggling and holding you back. You have all the resources now, so it's a case of implementing them gradually at your own pace. If you really want it, it will come. Trust in the process of life and make the most of it; decide to be that person who you want to be, because you can!

The Break-Out Zone (75–100)

You're still breaking out but doing a brilliant job of doing everything it takes to get there. You are clearly reaching new heights. Keep going and pushing forward. You know exactly what you need to do and sometimes the rest just takes time and the relevant experiences to reach zone zero or precisely where you want to be. On which note, enjoy the journey and know, at your deepest core level, that you'll get your outcome, irrespective of anyone or anything in your way. Ensure you keep being determined and tenacious about that!

Zone Zero (101 +)

Congratulations! You now know exactly what you want and have no hesitation in doing it and whatever else it takes to get it. Go for it and enjoy!

Now you can go back and look over the markers of a zone-zero personality at the end of Chapter Five to see how many more you feel you exhibit.

The Action List

Whatever your score may be this time round, it can be useful to further ask yourself the following questions again to assist you in forming an action list of all the things you need to do or areas you may wish to work on and release to advance where you want to be:

Key Questions

- Why did you give the answers you gave and what specifically were you referring to?
- What did you discover was different about yourself in comparison to when you last took the test?
- What does this reveal to you?
- What might you need to release, let go of, do or learn?
- What can you positively learn from your zone answers and score?
- How exactly can you push things forward?
- What is the key that will make the difference for you?
- Are you now ready to continue expanding your comfort zone boundaries, ambitions and desires even further?
- Are you eagerly anticipating the full discovery of where you want to go and constantly learning more about yourself, igniting new fresh purposes and intentions to keep things exciting?
- And if the answer to the last two questions is "no":
- Why not? What does this mean and what's the real root that needs addressing here?
- dIf you answered "yes" with much certainty, on the other hand, that's great stuff! Who knows where this may take you; no doubt somewhere you didn't ever consciously imagine. That's exactly when being able to trust in yourself and in the process of life is exciting.

"Insist that life begins at the end of your comfort zone!"

Summary

- Retaking the Zone Test is aimed at revealing a contrast with your first score, now you have worked through and applied the resources in this book.
- Recognizing your positive changes and anything that is left for you to work on will help you to push even further forward, whatever your new zone level is, as you develop throughout your life, discovering new purpose.
- Completing the action list and further introspective questioning of your answers will help with this.
- You can keep taking the Zone Test as many times as you like and use it as a tool to keep evolving and developing in whatever you wish.

CHAPTER TEN

THE FINAL WORD

A s we know, the one single reason for staying inside our comfort zone, not pushing boundaries and never really ever getting what we want ultimately comes down to fear, whether or not we are conscious of this.

So, to get anywhere we want to be, we must remove the fear and the blockages of energy stopping us. We must be masters at recognizing our fears and their derivatives that add up to our limitations; and at letting these go so we can move forward.

It's at this point when all memories and experiences become wisdom and allow for us to have no boundaries and create the space to carry ourselves forward, no matter how uncomfortable this may be at times. The point at which we are fully able to trust in the process of life; we can deal with anything.

And above even all that, there are three crucial elements:

1. When it comes to it, we are all far more resilient than we think we are, because we can and will handle whatever we're faced with. Therefore, there's no point worrying about it. Rather understand it and learn to trust in yourself!
2. Whenever you allow for new opportunities, pushing those boundaries and letting go of irrational fear, the universe responds accordingly and opens endless doors of infinite possibilities.
3. Always believe and know that, deep down at your core, you can be confident that no matter what happens along your journey, it's the right thing to guide you on your path to where you want to be and expect to be.

Just imagine, if I hadn't always had a strong core blueprint for myself, steering me to take certain bold decisions years ago to completely change the direction of my own life, you might not have been reading this book right now – and who knows what else as a consequence.

- The moment any of us make those wholehearted decisions to change things, be that overall or specifically in terms of moving toward the ultimate mission, be it personally or professionally, our life will change accordingly.
- Simply because every time you make that decision to step outside your comfort zone and determine your internal reality, you'll change the way you feel and act, changing your personality and therefore your external reality with the results you get. You'll change the quantum field around you and attract a different way of life, in line with the new you that you've created.
- Remember nothing is really real other than your perception; what you think and determine. We all create our own reality.

Essentially, everything is relative: nothing ventured, nothing gained – or, as I prefer to say, everything ventured, everything gained. It's another classic but all the same true: if we put more in, we'll certainly get more out.

So, the last questions at this point in the book are:

- If (God forbid) you died tomorrow, would you go out in a blaze of glory?
- What would your legacy be – what would you be remembered for?
- Would you feel happy leaving this existence knowing that you embraced life as we know it, and did all you could as you'd like? OR
- Would you be left pretty depressed at the thought of having lived a life of fear and regrets?

Above all else I sincerely hope to have assisted you in positively changing the perception and experience of what fear means to you, and your redefining of this, enabling you to release it once and for all and fully go for it, remembering always that:

What one person can do, so can another . . . if they make that deep-seated decision to apply the right mindset, and allow for the possibility.

Oh and . . .

Fortune really does favour the brave. Ultimately, it's well worth losing all those needless fears, inhibitions and limitations that are keeping you in your comfort zone; if you do, you can break out and live a life beyond limits!

SORTING ANY BUMPS IN THE ROAD

—————————

What Do I Do if I Still Feel the Same? Keep going! Sometimes things take time to integrate on an unconscious level – and that's where change really happens.

It's also important to check on your intentions for something: are these really right for you and are you focused on doing what you're doing in a positive context rather than in spite of something? Whatever you are wanting to do, do it for the right reasons, and ultimately for you, because you want to and can do.

In addition, ensure that you wholeheartedly believe you can do it! If you don't, it's worth exploring any deeply buried limitations that may be blocking you, all of which relate to some negative emotions born out of something. Keep going over the book; the answers are there, and something somewhere will click.

What If I Just Have No Motivation?

It's important to work out the real root of any lack of motivation. Firstly, is it superficial? Is it temporary? Could you be exhausted and experiencing burnout?

If that's the case, rest and break your routine as much as you can. Ideally have a complete change of scenery - take some time out or time off if you can and do something totally different. I know from personal experience that it has sometimes taken coming far away from things to spark some motivation in me. Even if it's something as simple as letting your hair down at a theme park for a day or two; some other kind of thrill-seeking activity, or a little getaway at the coast to chill out and blow the cobwebs away, it can make a big difference. A change is as good as a rest! It can help to spend some time meditating too as this aids rest, thinking space and creativity.

It may also be the case that you are experiencing a form of depression, anxiety disorder or even a physical condition; many of these can have symptoms such as a lack of motivation. So it might be worth a routine medical check.

Finally, perhaps your lack of motivation is explicable by the fact that whatever you are intending to do just isn't compelling enough for you. Perhaps you know deep down it's futile or not what you really want. If you think it's the latter, go over the life discovery model again and revisit Chapters Seven and Eight to keep learning more about yourself and exploring your core values. It could be the case that you need to align exactly what you want with what really gives you a spark and motivation.

What If There's No Change Despite Thinking Differently?

If you aren't seeing – or more importantly feeling – a change yet, you may need to give things a little longer to integrate and simply trust in the process. Perhaps change is occurring, but you just don't see it consciously yet.

Also, if change really isn't happening yet, it may mean that you don't really believe it at your deepest core. To help with this, check in on your blueprint and your unconscious mind; if whatever you do and whatever you think you want doesn't align with your core blueprint, things won't change, because you don't deep-down want them to. Keep reading through the book and applying anything relevant; the answers are there and you will find them when you are ready to, in line with your law of attraction.

I Feel Like I've Tried Everything, but Things Aren't Working

Breaking boundaries to step out of your current comfort zone isn't designed to be easy, otherwise it wouldn't even be a challenge in the first place, and no one would ever have any problems or limitations. It can however, be made simple.

Avoid overcomplicating it and certainly avoid overthinking it. If you do the necessary work, decide wholeheartedly and have full conviction behind what you are doing, then it's often a case of: just needing to stop trying so hard, believe, let things be and trust in yourself and the process of life.

Upon reaching this point it is likely that things will fully integrate and change will occur when you least expect it.

Have a go at the path of least resistance (less intensity or obsession and more trust, belief and expectation), if you have the key ingredients in place – it might well be what you are missing.

You may also need to explore strategies to find those that work best for you, depending on what you are doing or what specifically isn't working. Sometimes it may be a case of needing a little professional help or support to implement things to get you going in the right direction. Gregory Bateson, a British anthropologist and social scientist well-known in the 1940s for his work in this field, once said: "Man cannot be his own psychotherapist for long"; meaning sometimes we all need an external check to be able to see the wood for the trees.

What If I Just Can't Do It When It Comes Down to It?

You're probably just not ready yet. Go back to the Zone Test and Chapters Two, Seven and Eight, but read them with more of a focus on setting your own challenges and looking at your wider purpose, and doing internal work.

It may also be that you need more objective help, in which case think about seeing a professional.

Finally, you will find that some methods work better for you than others. Experiment with finding what works best for you and keep going! If you want it badly enough, you'll get it.

At a Glance

The six fundamentals needed to overcome fear and achieve everything you want:

- Know your true purpose, intention and outcome.
- Strong self-awareness to access your core roots with an absence of panic.
- Positive focus and attitude – everything you "can" do.
- A deep-seated belief in what you are doing and what you will do – be convinced!
- Trust yourself and trust the process of life.
- Practise, and enjoy the process – you become what you believe!

"You already have all the resources you'll ever need –
you just need to be open to seeing them."

RESOURCES AND REFERENCES

Please note: this section is designed to offer some useful resources for you to draw on and will give you a sense of where to start looking. Not all of the recommendations are mine personally – I always recommend that you do your own research and find what works best for you.

Useful Organizations

ABNLP – American Board of Hypnotherapy and Neuro Linguistic Programming (www.abh-abnlp.com). Lists NLP practitioners in the United States.

ANLP – Association for Neuro Linguistic Programming (www.anlp.org). This organization offers a list of certified NLP practitioners in the UK.

ADAA – Anxiety and Depression Association of America (https://adaa.org). Internationally provides education, training and support within the field of depression and anxiety.

Anxiety UK (www.anxietyuk.org.uk). A UK-based charity providing support for those affected by anxiety disorders.

CNHC – Complementary and Natural Healthcare Council (www.cnhc.org.uk). Official UK voluntary register of complementary healthcare practitioners.

Dsedtsy.com – A helpful information site and merchandise store to encourage you to do the things that scare you most and live life to the max.

Dr-em.co.uk – Useful resource, information and practice contact site.

Dr Joe Dispenza (drjoedispenza.com). Excellent video courses, and recorded seminars and live events information to attend regarding everything from health and healing to life in general.

GHR–General Hypnotherapy Register (www.general-hypnotherapy -register.com). This register lists practitioners within the field of hypnotherapy.

Interactive and Introspective Resources

Intuition Indicator™: https://intuitionindicator.questionpro.com
Personality indicator is: https://www.mbtionline.com
The Secret – watchdocumentaries.com/the-secret
The Zone Test™: https://zonetest.questionpro.com
What the Bleep Do We Know!? – http://whatthebleep.com

References

1   "When the brain knows no fear: Fear discovery could lead to new interventions for PTSD." *Current Biology*, University of Iowa, 16 December 2010, https:// www.sciencedaily.com/releases/2010/12/101216122006.htm

2   Kasian S.J., Owens J.E., Marsh G.R., "Binaural auditory beats affect vigilance, performance and mood", abstract (January 1998), Department of Psychiatry, Duke University Medical Center, Durham, North Carolina, USA. jdlane@acpub.duke.edu, Lane JD1, https://www.ncbi.nlm.nih.gov/pubmed/ 9423966

3   "Meditation offers significant heart benefits. It helps reduce stress and anxiety, which can lower heart rate and blood pressure while reducing harmful hormones." Harvard Medical School, August 2013. https://www. health. harvard.edu/heart-health/meditation-offers-significant-heart-benefits

4   Visualization Case1971 by Dr. O. Carl Simonton, a radiologist at the University of Texas. https://www.youtube.com/watch?v=b_Vh4qk6_BI

5   Norman Cousins, *Head First: The Biology of Hope*. New York: Dutton, 1989.

6   "An epidemiologic perspective on social anxiety disorder." Stein M.B., *J. Clin. Psychiatry* 2006; 67 suppl 12 3–8.
    Hedaya R., *Understanding Biological Psychiatry*. New York, N.Y W.W Norton & Company, 1996. pp 100–204.

7   A clinical research study from Japan, linking the levels of vitamin B6 and iron in the blood to the incidence of anxiety.
    http://healthlivingsolution.com/vitamin-b-iron-deficiency-can-cause -anxiety-panic-attacks/#ixzz4zwTxgfzQ

8   Tumours that can produce adrenaline and can cause anxiety
    https://www.healthline.com/health/pheochromocytoma

9   More information about the symptoms of Wilson's disease
    http://www.rightdiagnosis.com/w/wilsons_disease/intro.htm

10 "Mind Over Matter: Mental Training Increases Physical Strength." Shackell, Erin M. and Standing, Lionel G., Bishop's University, 2007: http:// west allen.typepad.com/brains_on_purpose/files/mind_over_matter_ shackell_07.pdf

11 Dr Michael Murray, Dr Joseph Pizzorno, Lara Pizzorno, *The Encyclopaedia of Healing Foods*, London: PIatkus, 2008. Ch. 4 p. 688.

12 The connection between B vitamins, depression and anxiety https://clinicaltrials.gov/ct2/show/NCT01672372

13 Locke and Latham's Goal Setting Theory Explained https://www.mindtools.com/pages/article/newHTE_87.htm

14 *The Gift: Poems by Hafiz*, London: Penguin Compass, 1999.

15 Research Article, "Mind-Set Matters Exercise and the Placebo Effect", alia Crum, J. and Langer, Ellen J., Association for Psychological Science, Harvard University, 2007: https://dash.harvard.edu/bitstream/handle/1/3196007/ Langer_ Exercise -PlaceboEffect.pdf?sequence=1

16 From the book, *Quantum Reality, Beyond the new physics*, Nick Herbert, 1985, Anchor Books, Ch.2, p.14.

17 Pao Chang, "What is Quantum Physics or Quantum Reality?", http://energyfanatics.com/2012/12/04/quantum-reality-exploring -universe-beyond-material-realm

Further Reading

Bandler, R. and Grinder J. Trance-formations: *Neuro-Linguistic Programming and the Structure of Hypnosis*. Boulder, CO : Real People Press, 1981.

Chopra, D. *Quantum Healing: Exploring the Frontiers of Mind-Body Medicine*. New York: Bantam Books, 1989.

Cousins, Norman. *Head First: The Biology of Hope*. New York: Dutton, 1989.

Hay, Louise. *You Can Heal Your Life*. Carlsbad, CA: Hay House, 1984.

Herbert, N. *Quantum Reality: Beyond the New Physic*s. New York: Anchor Books, 1985.

James, T. and W. Woodsmall. *Time Line Therapy and The Basis of Personality*. *Soquel*, CA: Meta Publications, 1988.

Kisen. *Yoga Pure and Simple*. Ebury Publishing, a division of Penguin Random House, London 2001.

Mardlin, E. *Mind Body Diabetes: A positive, powerful and proven solution to stop diabetes once and for all*. Forres: Findhorn Press, 2016.

Murray, M.T., J. Pizzorno and L. Pizzorno. *The Encyclopaedia of Healing Foods*. New York: Atria Books, a division of Simon & Schuster, 2005.

Pert, C.B. *Molecules of Emotion: Why You Feel the Way You Feel*. New York: Simon and Schuster, 1997.

Rossi. E. *The Psycho-Biology of Mind-Body Healing*. New York: W. W. Norton and Company, Inc, 1986.

Stein MB, *An epidemiologic perspective on social anxiety disorder*. J. Clin. Psychiatry 2006.

ABOUT THE AUTHOR

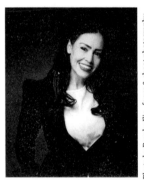

Photo by Branka Ilic, focus & shoot photography

Emma Mardlin, Ph.D., is renowned for her distinguished results in helping people achieve what others have deemed impossible. As a consultant therapist and performance coach holding a Ph.D. in psychotherapy, mind–body medicine, she implements a unique and holistic approach in all areas of her work.

Dr Em is founding partner of the Pinnacle Practice, a health and well-being clinic and training consultancy in London, Harley Street and Nottingham. In Practice, Em sees both adults and children with a host of life challenges from psychological and physical health concerns and severe traumas, to people in need of general life support from personal evolution to professional performance to get the very best outcomes in life.

Alongside this, Em integrates her metaphysical research work to reverse both psychological and physical health conditions, including the current reversal of two personal chronic health conditions, using herself as the primary lab rat.

Em further writes, lectures and provides professional courses and qualifications within her field for public organizations, government departments and private companies in the UK and United Arab Emirates. She also writes professionally for numerous journals and media.

Known for her warm nature, infectious positivity and humorous manner, Em sees the overcoming of her past adversities merely as valuable experiences to better help others.

For further information you can visit: www.dr-em.co.uk